I0066138

Immunogenetics

Edited by Nima Rezaei

Published in London, United Kingdom

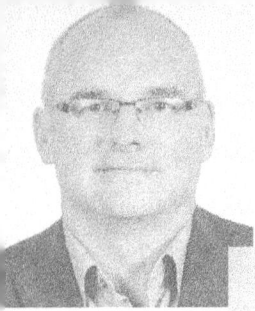
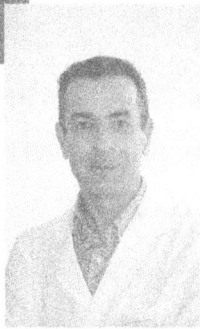
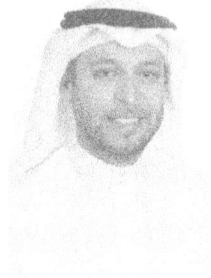
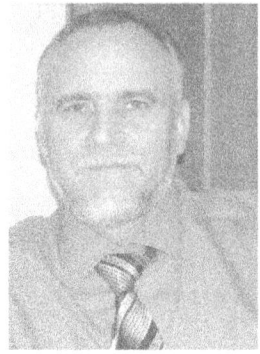
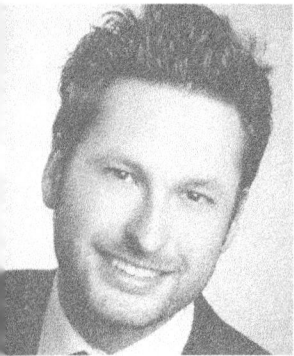
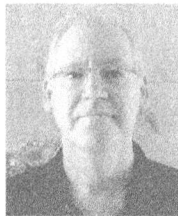
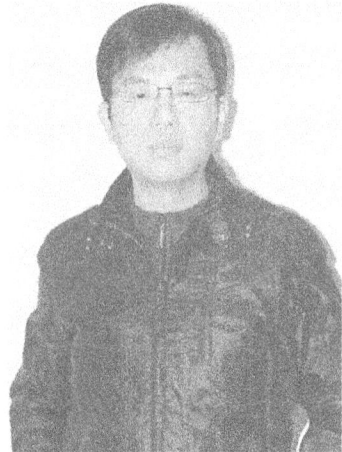

IntechOpen

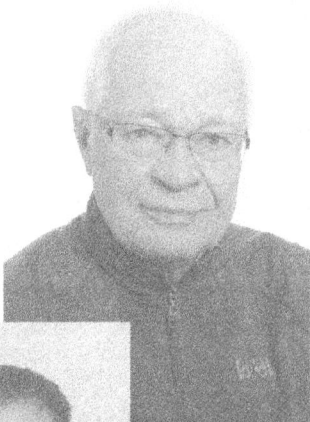
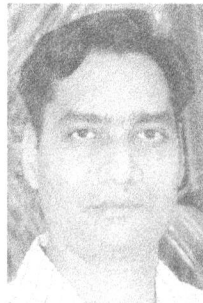
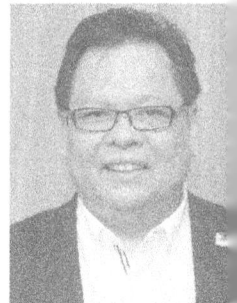
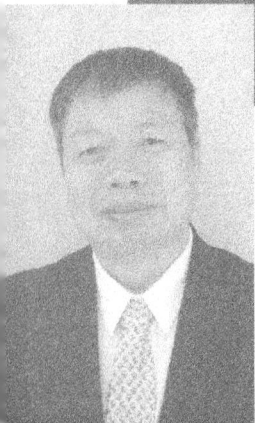
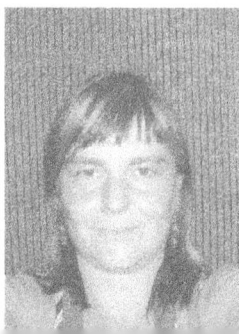
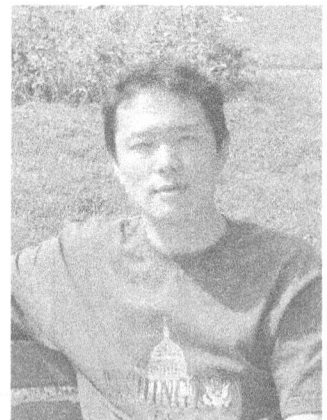

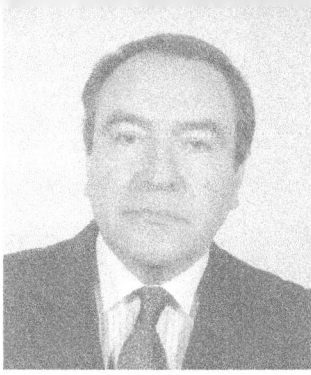

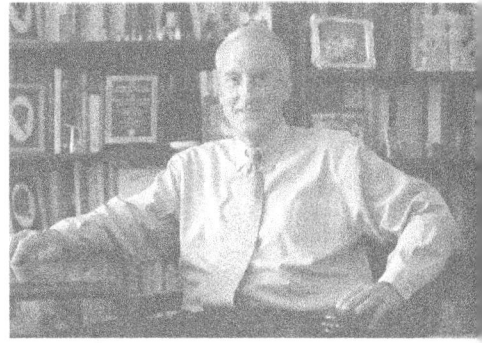

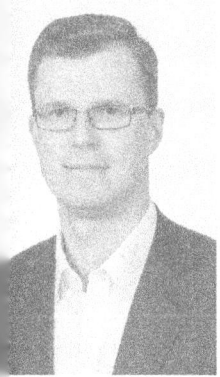

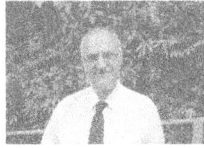

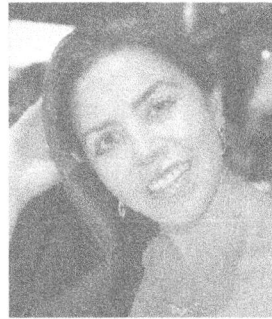

Supporting open minds since 2005

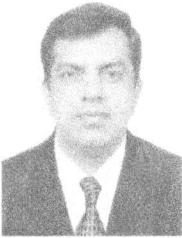

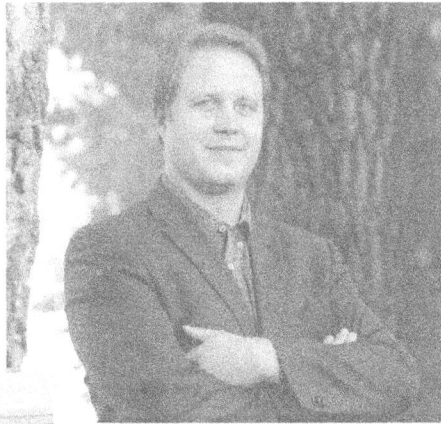

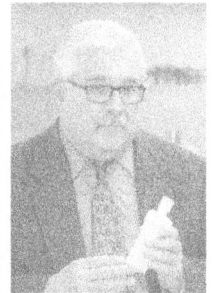

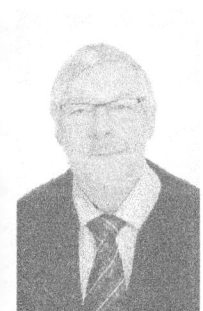

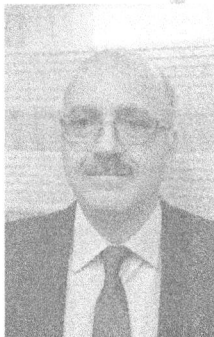

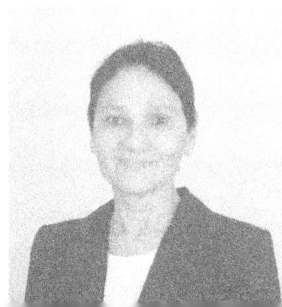

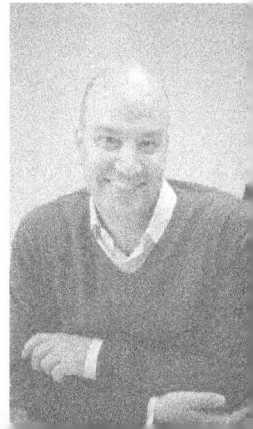

Immunogenetics
http://dx.doi.org/10.5772/intechopen.75838
Edited by Nima Rezaei

Contributors

Emilia Manole, Ionela Daniela Popescu, Carolina Constantin, Simona Mihai, Gisela Gaina, Elena Codrici, Alexandra Bastian, Monica Neagu, Christina Bade-Doeding, Funmilola Heinen, Gia-Gia Toni Ho, Florian Stieglitz, Rainer Blasczyk, Ramaprabhu Vempati, Gloria Guillermina Guerrero Manriquez, Nima Rezaei, Amene Saghazadeh

© The Editor(s) and the Author(s) 2019
The rights of the editor(s) and the author(s) have been asserted in accordance with the Copyright, Designs and Patents Act 1988. All rights to the book as a whole are reserved by INTECHOPEN LIMITED. The book as a whole (compilation) cannot be reproduced, distributed or used for commercial or non-commercial purposes without INTECHOPEN LIMITED's written permission. Enquiries concerning the use of the book should be directed to INTECHOPEN LIMITED rights and permissions department (permissions@intechopen.com).
Violations are liable to prosecution under the governing Copyright Law.

[(cc) BY]

Individual chapters of this publication are distributed under the terms of the Creative Commons Attribution 3.0 Unported License which permits commercial use, distribution and reproduction of the individual chapters, provided the original author(s) and source publication are appropriately acknowledged. If so indicated, certain images may not be included under the Creative Commons license. In such cases users will need to obtain permission from the license holder to reproduce the material. More details and guidelines concerning content reuse and adaptation can be found at http://www.intechopen.com/copyright-policy.html.

Notice
Statements and opinions expressed in the chapters are these of the individual contributors and not necessarily those of the editors or publisher. No responsibility is accepted for the accuracy of information contained in the published chapters. The publisher assumes no responsibility for any damage or injury to persons or property arising out of the use of any materials, instructions, methods or ideas contained in the book.

First published in London, United Kingdom, 2019 by IntechOpen
IntechOpen is the global imprint of INTECHOPEN LIMITED, registered in England and Wales, registration number: 11086078, The Shard, 25th floor, 32 London Bridge Street
London, SE19SG – United Kingdom
Printed in Croatia

British Library Cataloguing-in-Publication Data
A catalogue record for this book is available from the British Library

Additional hard copies can be obtained from orders@intechopen.com

Immunogenetics
Edited by Nima Rezaei
p. cm.
Print ISBN 978-1-83880-347-6
Online ISBN 978-1-83880-348-3
eBook (PDF) ISBN 978-1-83881-110-5

We are IntechOpen,
the world's leading publisher of
Open Access books
Built by scientists, for scientists

4,200+
Open access books available

116,000+
International authors and editors

125M+
Downloads

Our authors are among the

151
Countries delivered to

Top 1%
most cited scientists

12.2%
Contributors from top 500 universities

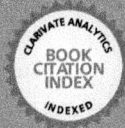

CLARIVATE ANALYTICS
BOOK
CITATION
INDEX
INDEXED

WEB OF SCIENCE™

Selection of our books indexed in the Book Citation Index
in Web of Science™ Core Collection (BKCI)

Interested in publishing with us?
Contact book.department@intechopen.com

Numbers displayed above are based on latest data collected.
For more information visit www.intechopen.com

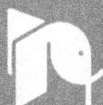

Meet the editor

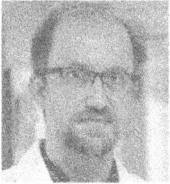

Professor Nima Rezaei gained his MD from Tehran University of Medical Sciences (TUMS) and subsequently obtained his MSc and PhD in Clinical Immunology and Human Genetics from the University of Sheffield, UK. He also spent a fellowship year in Pediatric Clinical Immunology and Bone Marrow Transplant at Newcastle General Hospital, UK. Professor Rezaei is now a full professor of Immunology and vice dean of International Affairs, School of Medicine, TUMS, and a cofounder and deputy president of the Research Center for Immunodeficiencies. He is also a founding president of the Universal Scientific Education and Research Network. Professor Rezaei has edited more than 20 international books, presented more than 400 lectures/posters in congresses/meetings, and published more than 700 articles in international scientific journals.

Contents

Preface

About 100 years ago, there was the very real fear of allograft rejection reactions when deciding on organ transplantation and blood transfusion. On facing this fear, scientists began to unravel the way tissue rejection occurs and find possible implications for its inhibition. The observation of excellence in tissue transplantation between identical twins suggested a genetic component to donor-recipient compatibility. Consequently, incompatibility of ABO blood groups—which are inherited—emerged as the fundamental factor for rejection reactions. This initial realization was among the first clues to the crossword of immunogenetics. However, the determining factor that yielded the fruit of immunogenetics dates back to the late twentieth century when human leukocyte antigen (HLA) molecules and genes controlling their expression were introduced as the heart of the allograft rejection problem. In this manner, immunity and genetics are closely linked with the discovery of hereditary varieties of immune responses.

The introductory chapter of *Immunogenetics* provides an overview of the most important implications of immunogenetics after a brief introduction to the HLA system and its immunological function.

Despite its initial rejection, the manuscript introducing Western blotting, also known as immunoblotting, was published in the early 1980s. Since then, the scientific community is still interested in adopting different Western blotting approaches to detect immunologic proteins in biological samples. The second chapter explores in detail the value of Western blotting as an immunoassay in today's world.

In addition to rejection reactions, HLA molecules expressed by tumor cells can drive tumor development and play a critical role in avoiding detection by the immune system. In Chapter 3, the dynamic interaction between immune escape mechanisms and HLA regulation is presented.

Psychoneuroimmunology is a discipline with roots that connect the brain, behavior, and immunity. Findings of immunogenetic abnormalities that influence neurocircuitry and behavior have made this field especially interesting. Chapter 4 is dedicated to reviewing such research.

Tuberculosis is a potentially serious global health problem caused by *Mycobacterium tuberculosis* (Mtb) in humans. Different immune cells, for example, macrophages, dendritic cells, neutrophils, and natural killer cells, are induced in response to Mtb infection. Genetic alteration of antituberculosis immune responses has been associated with predisposition to different forms of tuberculosis. The last chapter discusses the immunogenetics of tuberculosis along with potential implications for immunotherapy.

We are very pleased to have had the opportunity to write this book on immunogenetics for IntechOpen, which is continuously attempting to open scientific minds by publishing open access books. We hope that this book has, though concisely, answered some immunogenetic questions.

Nima Rezaei
Tehran University of Medical Sciences,
Tehran, Iran

Chapter 1

Introductory Chapter: Immunogenetics

Amene Saghazadeh and Nima Rezaei

1. Major histocompatibility complex (MHC): the master system for self-/nonself-recognition

It is a gene family found in many vertebrates. In humans, the "HLA" is interchangeably used with MHC. The MHC gene family is composed of three main subfamilies clustered near one another on chromosome 6. As shown in **Figure 1**, MHC class III genes space between MHC class I and class II genes. Glycoproteins encoded by MHC class I genes are present on the surface of all nucleated somatic cells, while the expression of MHC II glycoproteins is largely restricted to the specialized antigen-presenting cells (APCs) such as dendritic cells, macrophages, and B cells. Both have extracellular domains that form the peptide-binding region. Those of MHC class I molecules govern the presentation of peptide (antigen) primarily derived from intracellular sources (endogenous) to $CD8^+$ cytotoxic T lymphocytes (CTLs), while those of MHC class II molecules are particularly effective at presentation of peptide primarily originated from extracellular sources (exogenous) to $CD4^+$ helper T (T_H) cells. In the following, the specific mechanisms of action appear:

2. MHC class I

T-cell receptor (TCR) on the surface of CTLs interacts with peptide-MHC class I complex. It has the ability to discriminate self from foreign. CTLs are stimulated upon TCR recognition of foreign peptides. Stimulated CTLs promote T-cell proliferation and lysis in peptide-pulsed target cells. Also MHC class I molecules interact with NK cell receptors, e.g., killer-immunoglobulin-like receptors (KIRs), thereby controlling effector functions of NK cells that can damage self-components, for example, cell cytotoxicity and excessive inflammation [1]. In this manner, MHC I molecules induce self-tolerance via a NK cell-dependent mechanism as well.

3. Class I MHC restriction of CTLs

Because both self and foreign peptides can bind to class I MHC molecules, so a question to ask is what would happen to class I MHC molecules loaded with self-peptide. The answer lies within the process by which T lymphocytes are selected in the thymus. Thereby, CTLs can enter circulation if their surface TCR is reactive to self-class I MHC molecules loaded with foreign, not self, peptides. This reaction is known as class I MHC restriction of CTLs, because it occurs only in the presence of self-class I MHC molecules (for review see [2]). As if, class I MHC molecules act as parent to CTLS. Two possibilities arise [3]. First, self-class I MHC compatibility is necessary for sensitizing of the foreign peptide and thereby for binding and lysis of the target cell

IntechOpen

900 Kb

DAXX
ZBTB22
TAPBP
RGL2
PFDN6
WDR46
B3GALT4

4000 Kb
3800 Kb
HLA-F

HLA-G

3600 Kb

800 Kb

RPS18
VPS52

4000
Kb

RING1
HSD17B8
SLC39A7
PRXB
COL11A2

3000 Kb
HLA-A

MHC-
I

6p21.3

HLA-E
2800 Kb

700 Kb

2000
Kb

HLA-DPB2
HLA-DPB1
HLA-DPA1
HLA-DOA

2200 Kb
HLA-C

600 Kb

MHC-
III

HLA-B
MICA

BRD2
HLA-DMA
HLA-DMB
HLA-Z

1000
Kb

2000 Kb

500 Kb

2000 Kb
TNF

PSMB9
TAP1
PSMB8
TAP2
HLA-DOB

MHC-
II

LST1

400 Kb

0
C6orf48

Chromosome 6

EHMT2
CFB
SKIV2L

HLA-DOB

HLA-DQB2
MIR3135B
HLA-DQA2
MTCO3P1

300 Kb

TNXB
NOTCH4
1000 Kb

HLA-DQB1
HLA-DQA1
HLA-DRB5

200 Kb

100 Kb

HLA-DRB5

HLA-DRB9
HLA-DRA

0

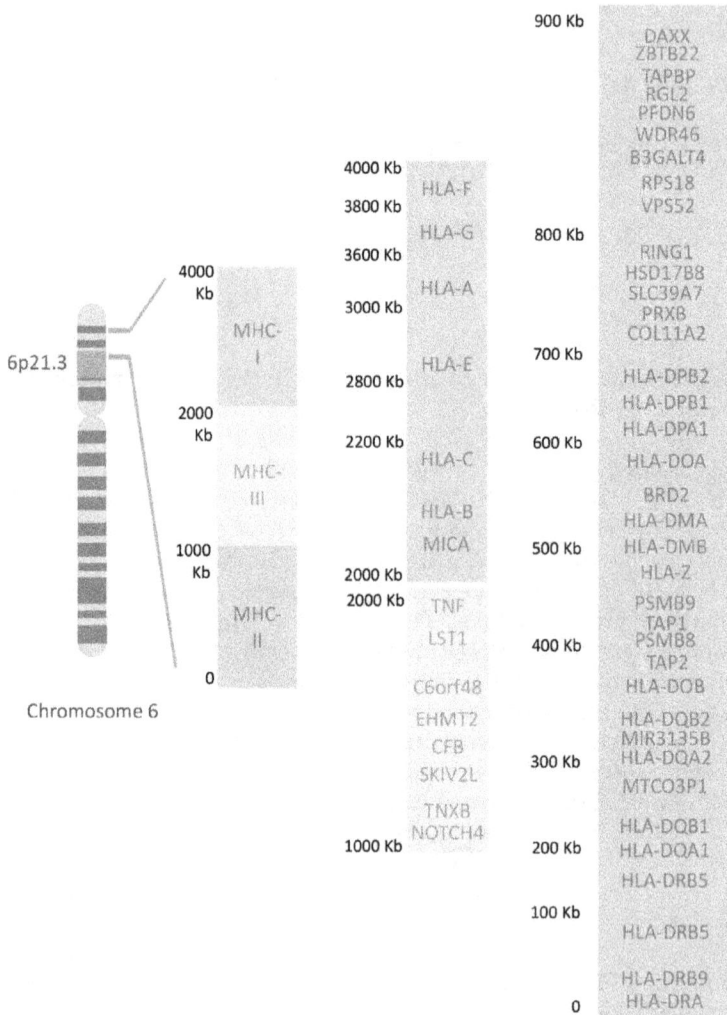

Figure 1.
The genetic architecture of human major histocompatibility complex (MHC).

by CTLs. In this case, there might be specific MHC gene products and the interactions between them that function to distinguish self from foreign. Second, self-components undergo changes in composition on encountering foreign antigen, so that their recognition is not possible unless a compatible class I MHC system is available.

4. MHC class II

4.1 Macrophages

Extracellular peptides or pathogens are engulfed by phagocytosis into macrophages and assembled into a vesicle, called phagosome. Lysosomes combine with the phagosome to digest substances in order to extract their antigens. MHC class II molecules orient antigens to the outer surface of cell membrane, where T_H cells stand ready to bind and assist with recognition of antigens. Recognition of a foreign antigen by T_H cells would force more macrophages to phagocyte pathogens.

4.2 B lymphocytes

Immunoglobulins are attached to the surface of B cells. Binding of a foreign antigen to these immunoglobulins induces the engulfment of that particular antigen by B cells. B cells prepare ingested antigen for presentation by MHC class II molecules. Peptide-MHC II complex would engage T_H cells that promote proliferation of antibody-producing plasma cells. Antibodies produced by plasma cells enter the circulation and form complex with matching antigens. Matching antigen-antibody complexes are susceptible to cleavage.

In this manner, MHC class I and class II molecules are very important in the initiation of cell-mediated and antibody-mediated immune responses. As a result, they have always been in the center of attention of immunogeneticists.

5. The genetic architecture of human MHC

Figure 1 shows three main MHC classes of genes. Occupying about 0.1% of the human genome [4], the MHC ranks as the most gene-dense region in the human genome. Two hundred and twenty-four MHC loci have been so far isolated from humans, among which 20–30% [5] are associated with a known or putative function in innate and adaptive immune responses [4], while the rest act as mediators of growth, development, mating, reproduction, odor, and olfaction [6]. This would imply that MHC is working on contextually different aspects of the evolution. As in mammalian genome, some MHC genes related to adaptive immune system are present in invertebrate genomes. This would tell us that the origin of the adaptive immune system dates back to at least 400 million years ago [7].

6. Evolution and selection of MHC polymorphisms

The MHC class I and class II genes continue as the most polymorphic genes in mammals. However, there are specific loci that exhibit a higher level of polymorphism compared with other loci studied in the same population. Mounting evidence supports that selective MHC polymorphisms might play a role in evolution, so that they will be maintained within one species or even command one species to be transformed into another [8]. Different hypotheses exist regarding profitable variations that are provided by MHC polymorphisms making them favorable to be accumulated by natural selection. For example, in the context of immunity, the overdominance hypothesis states that individuals being heterozygous for those certain MHC polymorphisms, the so-called extraordinary polymorphisms, will have an advantage over the homozygous individuals that the MHC function is more powerful in terms of types of peptides that they can bind to and recognition of more peptide types, in turn, would mean protection against a broader range of pathogens. This is known as heterozygous advantage or overdominance selection. For more information regarding other hypotheses, please see [2, 9–12].

7. Challenges in mapping MHC genes

MHC loci are difficult to map due to a number of reasons including:

1. There are many sequences and structural variations that can be extracted from MHC.

2. There is strong linkage disequilibrium between different loci that can influence the accuracy of analysis of the immunogenetic data.

3. There are nonadditive effects within the MHC loci and also epistatic interactions between the MHC and other genes that are able to affect total genomic variance [4].

As detailed in [5], different approaches have been developed for sequencing the MHC and discovery of potential copy-number variation (CNV) and of SNP regions. Sanger sequencing combined with next-generation DNA sequencing technologies can be used to detect SNPs, describe their characteristics, and obtain information for haplotype phasing.

Serological techniques and solid-phase immunoassays offer HLA typing with an appropriate resolution [13]. However, it is noteworthy to mention that despite about one century of effort, HLA (class I and II) typing—which is used to match donor and recipient for transplantation of the stem cells, cord blood, and kidney—might be challenging for bioinformaticians in some instances. Therefore, external proficiency testing (EPT) is performed to resolve ambiguities in HLA typing. According to a report of the Ad-Hoc Committee of the American Society for Histocompatibility and Immunogenetics, there is no need to resolve all ambiguous results [14]. The committee recommends that if there is more than one possible HLA genotype at the time of clinical decision-making, then we only need to refer to the criteria of EPT, which is attached to a list of common and well-documented (CWD) HLA alleles. For each HLA locus, e.g., HLA-A, HLA-B, HLA-C, HLA-DRB1, HLA-DQB1, HLA-DRB3/4/5, HLA-DQA1, and HLA-DPB1, CWD alleles consist of about 27–47% of the total alleles.

8. The international ImMunoGeneTics information system

For almost 30 years, the international ImMunoGeneTics (IMGT) information system has been made available free on http://imgt.cines.fr. IMGT is composed of immunogenetic information on sequences, nucleotides, genes and their polymorphisms, and proteins of the immune system including immunoglobulins or antibodies, TCR, and MHC. It can be useful for diagnostic, therapeutic, and engineering purposes and also research in the different fields of medicine, in particular, autoimmune diseases, infectious diseases, acquired immunodeficiency syndrome (AIDS), and blood cancers. In this manner, IMGT helps operationalize the continuum between specialist and generalist databases.

9. Immunogenetics and inherited risk of multifactorial diseases

9.1 HLA loci

Genetic studies have provided evidence for association of loci on HLA and:

1. Autoimmune and inflammatory diseases: acute anterior uveitis, alopecia areata, asthma, atopic dermatitis, eczema, rheumatoid arthritis, Behçet's disease, celiac disease, collagenous colitis, granulomatosis with polyangiitis (Wegener granulomatosis), generalized vitiligo, IgA nephropathy, primary biliary cirrhosis, psoriasis, ankylosing spondylitis, systemic lupus erythematosus, vasculitis, type 1 diabetes, Crohn's disease, ulcerative colitis, dermatomyositis, and Graves' disease

2. Infections: human immunodeficiency virus (HIV) set-point viral load (spVL), HIV-1 control, acquired immunodeficiency syndrome (AIDS) progression, chronic hepatitis B infection and viral clearance, hepatitis B, hepatitis B and C virus-related hepatocellular carcinoma, hepatitis B-related liver cirrhosis, chronic hepatitis C infection, human papillomavirus (HPV) seropositivity, dengue shock syndrome, leprosy, *M. tuberculosis* infection, malaria, resistance to enteric fever, and visceral leishmaniasis

3. Gastrointestinal diseases: Barrett's esophagus

4. Neurological disorders: Parkinson's disease, narcolepsy, juvenile myoclonic epilepsy, spinocerebellar ataxia, myasthenia gravis, and multiple sclerosis

5. Psychiatric disorders: schizophrenia and autism

6. Joint diseases: knee osteoarthritis

7. Cancers of the nasopharynx, cervix, colorectum, lung, blood cells, and bone marrow (lymphoid cancers)

8. Adverse drug reactions: Stevens-Johnson syndrome/toxic epidermal necrolysis (carbamazepine), agranulocytosis (clozapine), pancreatitis (thiopurine), and liver injury (terbinafine, fenofibrate, ticlopidine, and pazopanib)

9. Response to vaccines: hepatitis B

10. Male infertility due to nonobstructive azoospermia

9.2 Non-HLA loci

Generally, loci on non-HLA genes are involved in genetic predisposition to a variety of autoimmune and inflammatory disorders, among which the most associated have been identified in three genes: cytotoxic T-lymphocyte-associated antigen 4 (CTLA4), protein tyrosine phosphatase (PTPN22), and tumor necrosis factor-α (TNF). In particular, it is noticeable that patients who receive hematopoietic stem cell transplantation (SCT) from matched sibling donor might develop acute graft-versus-host disease (GVHD). This reflects that non-HLA components have a part in making the immunogenetic profile that needs special attention in patients scheduled to undergo stem cell transplantation.

10. Immunogenetics and the spectrum of immune disorders

By engaging pattern recognition receptors (PRRs)—including Toll-like receptors (TLRs) and nucleotide-binding oligomerization domain-like receptors (NLRs)—and signal-transducing molecules, e.g., interleukin-1 receptor-associated kinase 4 (IRAK4), the innate immune system forms the center of recognition of molecular patterns and therefore the first line of defense against foreign antigens. Abnormally low activity of this system causes underdetection of foreign agents that makes individuals susceptible to being infected, while the unwanted action of this system is being reactive to self-components, which is seen in autoimmune situations. In this manner, if anything hinders the proper functioning of the immune system, for example, genetic factors, then it is most likely that the body is prone to autoimmune and infectious diseases.

Immunogenetics aims to cover HLA and non-HLA effects for all the aforementioned categories with emphasis on autoimmune disorders and infections, two ends of the spectrum of immune disorders.

11. Autoimmune diseases

11.1 Psoriasis

Psoriasis was initially known as a disease of abnormal keratinocyte proliferation presented with chronic plaque in the majority of instances that can predispose patients to cardiovascular, psychiatric, and joint complications. It is already considered an immune-mediated skin disease where both innate and adaptive immunities play a role in initiating psoriatic lesions. Of note, Th1 pathway is overstimulated; there are high levels of Th1 cytokines and chemokines including IL-2, IL-12, and IFN-γ in psoriatic plaques. T cells, natural killer cells, natural killer T cells, and, to a lesser extent, neutrophils contribute to cutaneous inflammation in psoriasis as well. More interestingly, dendritic cells through antigen presentation to T cells can lead to plaque formation.

Consistent with its different clinical facets, there is a catalog consisting more than 60 loci identified as risk genes for psoriasis. In particular, the risk allele at MHC class I gene is present in about half of patients with psoriasis. Generally, HLA and non-HLA genetic loci associated with psoriasis are important mediators of antigen presentation, Th17/IL-23 axis, T-cell function, antiviral immunity, macrophage activation, and nuclear factor-κB (NF-κB)-dependent signaling. A simple mechanism for these genetic risk alleles in pathogenesis of psoriasis is likely to be mediated through reducing the threshold for activation of the innate immunity.

11.2 Rheumatoid arthritis (RA)

RA is a chronic inflammatory disease of synovial joints characterized by synovial hyperplasia, production of autoantibodies such as rheumatoid factor (RF) and anti-citrullinated protein antibody (ACPA), bone deformity, and systemic manifestations. Collectively, RA is associated with unfavorable long-term prognosis. Different cells such as macrophages, monocytes, fibroblasts, and T cells act to make an orchestra of cytokines, e.g., IL-1, IL-6, and TNF-α, which are central to the abnormal signaling pathways underlying this inflammatory arthritis.

RA has a long-recognized association with alleles at MHC class II gene that contain a common amino acid sequence in the HLA-DRB1 region, e.g., HLA-DRB1*0404 and DRB1*0401. In addition, there are non-HLA genetic loci associated with RA in ACPA-positive patients. As reviewed in [15], RA-associated genes are known to play a role in the nuclear factor-κB (NF-κB)-dependent signaling, TCR signaling, and JAK-STAT signaling.

11.3 Autoimmune thyroid diseases (AITDs)

As for other autoimmune disorders, AITDs such as Graves's disease and Hashimoto's thyroiditis are of T-cell-mediated autoimmune disorders mainly characterized by production of autoantibodies against and T-cell infiltration in the thyroid gland. Thereby, the immune system cannot correctly maintain a constant battle causing the gland to malfunction, which can be manifested as hyper- or hypothyroidism. Generally, AITDs are of special importance in practice because of their comorbidities with other autoimmune diseases.

Among risk alleles for AITDs are genetic variants associated with thyroid function. However, a variety of AITDs-related genetic loci occur within immune-modulating and HLA genes, which are known to contribute to peripheral tolerance, T-lymphocyte activation, and antigen presentation. In this manner, a mechanism of immunogenetic susceptibility to AITDs is maintained through interference with central and peripheral tolerance, APCs, and subsequent activation of T cells.

11.4 Primary biliary cirrhosis (PBC)

It is a disease of small intrahepatic bile ducts regarded as an autoimmune liver disease with the presence of the antimitochondrial antibody (AMA) in all except a minority of patients (up to 10%). Supporting this is that the infiltration of auto-reactive CD4+ T cells and CD8+ T cell specific to AMA has increased manifold in the liver of patients with PBS. T cells along with other immune cells such as B cells, macrophages, eosinophils, and natural killer cells take part in the composition of the portal inflammation. Eventually, such a chronic inflammation would progress to the loss of biliary epithelial cells.

Genetic studies have detected HLA variants conferring susceptibility to PBC. However, there were HLA variants that seemed protective against PBC. Non-HLA loci associated with PBC mainly involve genes associated with T cells. In particular, they contribute to IL-12-JAK-STAT4, CD80/CD86, and IL7R-α/CD127 signaling pathways, which are known to play a role in Th1 T-cell polarization, TCR signaling, and T-cell homeostasis, respectively. Other PBC-associated non-HLA loci are related to B-cell function, TNF signaling, and NF-κB signaling.

11.5 Type 1 diabetes mellitus (T1DM)

T1DM is a T-cell-mediated autoimmune disorder characterized by the presence of autoantibodies against islet cells. Increasing incidence of T1DM and its potential microvascular and macrovascular complications have shed light on the need for identifying more effective prevention strategies and new treatment targets. To this end, it is essential to enhance our understanding of the pathogenesis of T1DM.

It is a polygenic disorder where the HLA class II genes account for almost half of genetic susceptibility for T1DM. Interestingly, there are loci of these genes that have also been associated with protection from T1DM. Of the so-far-identified non-HLA genes are a variable number of tandem mini-satellite repeats (VNTR) and CTLA-4.

11.6 Systemic lupus erythematosus (SLE)

It is a chronic autoimmune disease affecting multiple organ systems includ-ing the skin, heart, blood, muscle and joints, kidneys, and lungs. As if, SLE is the winner of all fights with the immune system that is not possible unless the immune tolerance against self-components is broken. Activation of innate immune responses and of inflammatory processes along with production of type I interfer-ons and autoantibodies favors pathogenesis of SLE, while mechanisms of clearance of immune complexes such as apoptosis, neutrophil extracellular traps (NET), and nucleic acid sensing are defective. In particular, evidence indicates the multifaceted role of neutrophils in SLE. Lupus neutrophils undergo epigenetic changes causing them to produce higher levels of cytokines that would induce T- and B-cell abnor-malities. Also, neutrophils directly contribute to the formation of NET, which is increased in SLE, while clearance of NET materials is impaired in SLE.

As expected, such a complex situation involves contribution by both HLA and non-HLA genes. Several HLA genes including HLA-DRB1, HLA-DQB2,

HLA-DQA2, and HLA-DR3 have been associated with susceptibility to SLE and with the autoantibody profile (anti-dsDNA, anti-Ro, and anti-La) in patients with SLE. Genes encoding interferon regulatory factors (IRFs), STAT4, IFIH1, and osteopontin (OPN) contribute to polygenic high IFN signatures, while TREX1, STING, SAMHD1, and TRAP are known to give rise to monogenic high IFN signatures in SLE. Monogenic SLE results from mutation(s) in genes related to classical complement pathway, apoptosis, and antinucleosome antibody production. SLE-associated genes that occur in regulatory regions (e.g., exons, splice sites, introns, and intergenic sites) are TNFAIP3, TNIP1, BLK, ETS1, PRDM1, and IKZF1. Finally, there are SNPs located within the coding region of genes PTPN22 and immunoglobulin-like transcript 3 receptor (ILT3) that have been linked with SLE.

11.7 Systemic sclerosis (SSc)

SSc is considered a complex multisystem disease characterized by a heterogeneous spectrum of clinical manifestations ranging from limited to diffuse cutaneous SSc. Both innate and adaptive immune systems, fibroblasts, and small vessels show abnormal function in SSc.

There is a long list of HLA genes conferring susceptibility to clinical and autoantibody subgroups of SSc. Also, some HLA genes appear to be protective of SSc. Non-HLA genes associated with SSc are known to play a role in innate immunity, interferon signature and inflammation, adaptive immune responses, B- and T-cell proliferation, survival and cytokine production, apoptosis, autophagy, and fibrosis.

12. Neurological diseases

There is sufficient evidence to support the immunogenetic basis for some neurological diseases, in particular, multiple sclerosis, Alzheimer's disease, Parkinson's disease, neuromyelitis optica, myasthenia gravis, and amyotrophic lateral sclerosis. Below provides a rapid overview of the immunogenetics of MS as the prototype of such neurological diseases.

12.1 Multiple sclerosis (MS)

It is the most common inflammatory disease of the CNS, which after interfering with normal myelination results in axonal degeneration. The pathologic characteristics of MS are demyelinating lesions, which can be broadly classified according to whether or not autoimmune processes precede demyelination. In this manner, there are lesions arising from T-cell-mediated and T-cell plus antibody-mediated autoimmune encephalomyelitis, while sometimes demyelination is an initial clue resulted from viruses and toxins. Generally, MS is considered a chronic autoimmune disease, which is primarily characterized by activation of $CD4^+$ autoreactive T cells and Th1 T-cell polarization and then by the production of antibodies, complement factors, and $CD8^+$ T cells damaging the CNS tissues.

Studies suggest a strong genetic component for MS; more than 100 genetic loci have been so far identified to confer MS susceptibility. HLA genes totally account for about 10% of the genetic variance of MS. In particular, MHC class II gene HLA-DRB1*1501 is present in about 50% of patients with MS. After that, the IL-7R-α chain gene can explain about 30% of all cases. Also, IL-2RA is another non-HLA gene implicated in MS. Fresh evidence emerged that supports the potential of KIR genes as a risk or protective factor in the immunogenetics of MS. Both CD4$^+$ T cells and NK cells express KIRs. CD4$^+$ T cells that express KIRs are involved in antibody production and NK cells that express KIRs mediate antiviral and antitumoral innate immune responses. Therefore, KIR polymorphisms can affect the individual's risk for MS through the impact they have on antiviral immunity and antibody production. Now there is a big hope for the future of pharmacogenomics of MS when the immunogenetic information may help to predict treatment response, but it is not fulfilled yet!

13. Infectious diseases

13.1 Human immunodeficiency virus (HIV)

There is a variable degree of immunity to HIV. Genetic factors account for about one-fourth of this variation, among which are HLA genes that through interaction with CD8$^+$ cytotoxic T and CD4$^+$ helper T cells help the initiation of anti-HIV adaptive immune responses, thereby conferring resistance to HIV. Studies have shown associations of HLA genes with accelerated disease progression, slow disease progression, protection against infection, reduced viral load levels, and increased susceptibility to infection. In addition, KIR genes have been implicated in resistance to HIV. More interesting is that the development of TB in people with HIV is, at least in part, determined by individual immunogenetic constitution.

13.2 Hepatitis B virus (HBV) and hepatitis C virus (HCV) infection

Infection with HBV or HCV influences the expression of intrahepatic genes, thereby leaving patients liable to chronic liver disease, cirrhosis, and hepatocellular carcinoma. Virus-specific T-cell responses are central to the removal of infected hepatocytes, and therefore, the kinetics of these responses can aid in monitoring clinical recovery. In 1 year, about 2% of patients with chronic HBV infection will experience spontaneous viral clearance, which is characterized by HBV-specific T cells temporary appearing in the peripheral blood. Such an experience does not occur at all in the case of chronic HCV.

Genetic factors contribute to interindividual variation in clinical course of HBV and HCV infection. GWASs have identified HLA and non-HLA that confer susceptibility to persistent HBV infection, progression of disease, and risk of HBV-related hepatocellular carcinoma. Again, both HLA and non-HLA genes have been linked with spontaneous clearance of HCV. Two genes MICA and DEPDC5 demonstrated association with HCV-related hepatocellular carcinoma.

13.3 Tuberculosis (TB)

Mycobacterium tuberculosis is recognized by innate immune receptors including TLRs, C-type lectin receptors (CLRs), and NLRs. Upon its recognition, different mechanisms by which immune cells (macrophages and T cells) and cytokines (IL-12, IFN-γ, IL-4, TNF-α, IL-10, IL-6, and TGF-β) can mediate antimycobacterial functions are engaged. Consistently, increasing evidence supports the individual genetic contribution to the control of tuberculosis infection, severe primary tuberculosis, and pulmonary tuberculosis. Genetic risk factors for developing TB include both HLA and non-HLA genes.

14. Immunogenetics and immunosenescence

Immunosenescence refers to immune decline with age, which causes increased infection risk and related morbidity and mortality in the elderly. It is characterized by a chronic low-grade inflammation that arises from aberrant innate and adaptive immune responses, playing a role in a myriad of diseases including, but not limited to, atherosclerosis, obesity, type 2 diabetes, osteoporosis, osteoarthritis, neurode-generative diseases, major depression, and malignancy. In the last four decades, immunosenescence has received great attention from geneticists. However, due to heterogeneous methodology, we are still unable to generalize the findings to all elderly people. In addition to HLA genes, non-HLA genes related to adaptive immunity and to innate immunity appear to contribute to the immunogenetic network of human longevity.

15. Immunogenetics of atopic diseases

The most common chronic diseases afflicting children are asthma, hay fever (allergic rhinitis), and eczema (atopic dermatitis). Due to their strong association with concurrent atopic dermatitis, both asthma and allergic rhinitis can be defined as a type of atopic diseases. In this manner, atopy can be used as an umbrella term that describes a group of diseases, e.g., asthma, allergic rhinitis, food allergy, and urticaria. Atopy is considered a result of a Th2-mediated process, where Th2 cytokines promote the production of IgE by IgE+ memory B cells and plasma cells.

Genome screens show that, in general, atopic diseases are largely heritable (60%) and suggest that shared genes for atopy and other autoimmune diseases lie on the short arm of chromosome 6 where MHC gene are. In particular, the airway epithelium undergoes changes in asthma, and as a result, common genes are likely to cause asthma and other epithelial-based diseases, e.g., Crohn's disease and psoriasis. In addition, genes encoding innate immune receptors and cytokines, which are central to the initiation and progression of allergic responses, contribute to the immunogenetic network of atopy.

16. Vaccinomics and adversomics: immunogenetics and response to vaccination

Immune responses to vaccines vary between individuals. The main goal of vaccinomics is to deal with genes that may explain a substantial part of this variation. For example, studies estimate the variation in antibody response to hepatitis B surface antigen (HBsAg), measles virus, mumps virus, and rubella virus to be about 60, 88, 38, and 45% hereditary based. Generally, HLA and non-HLA genes encoding cytokines, cell surface receptors, and TLRs affect immune responses to vaccines, e.g., HBV, smallpox, MMR, and seasonal influenza. Moreover, there is evidence that genetic factors play a role in determining vaccine safety and adverse events, and consequently, it led to the emergence of adversomics. Overall, vaccinomics and adversomics facilitate prediction of vaccine efficacy and safety by using immunogenetic knowledge, and this in itself helps in developing more effective vaccines.

In this manner, *immunogenetics* aims to specify situations in which genetic mutations cause the immune system to be functionally imperfect and secure solutions for them.

Acknowledgements

We apologize to all colleagues whose excellent works could not be cited due to space constraints.

Author details

Amene Saghazadeh[1] and Nima Rezaei[2,3,4*]

1 Systematic Review and Meta-analysis Expert Group (SRMEG), Universal Scientific Education and Research Network (USERN), Tehran, Iran

2 Research Center for Immunodeficiencies, Children's Medical Center, Tehran University of Medical Sciences, Tehran, Iran

3 Department of Immunology, School of Medicine, Tehran University of Medical Sciences, Tehran, Iran

4 Network of Immunity in Infection, Malignancy and Autoimmunity (NIIMA), Universal Scientific Education and Research Network (USERN), Tehran, Iran

*Address all correspondence to: rezaei_nima@yahoo.com

IntechOpen

© 2019 The Author(s). Licensee IntechOpen. This chapter is distributed under the terms of the Creative Commons Attribution License (http://creativecommons.org/licenses/by/3.0), which permits unrestricted use, distribution, and reproduction in any medium, provided the original work is properly cited. (cc) BY

References

[1] Kim S et al. Licensing of natural killer cells by host major histocompatibility complex class I molecules. Nature. 2005;**436**(7051):709-713

[2] Hughes AL, Yeager M. Natural selection at major histocompatibility complex loci of vertebrates. Annual review of genetics. 1998;**32**(1):415-435

[3] Zinkernagel RM, Doherty PC. Immunological surveillance against altered self-components by sensitised T lymphocytes in lymphocytes choriomeningitis. Nature. 1974;**251**(5475):547

[4] Matzaraki V et al. The MHC locus and genetic susceptibility to autoimmune and infectious diseases. Genome Biology. 2017;**18**(1):76

[5] Christiansen FT, Tait BD. Immunogenetics: Methods and Applications in Clinical Practice. Humana Press; 2012

[6] Penn DJ, Ilmonen P. Major Histocompatibility Complex (MHC): Human. eLS; 30 May 2001

[7] Consortium MHCS. Complete sequence and gene map of a human major histocompatibility complex. Nature. 1999;**401**:921-923

[8] Klein J, Sato A, Nikolaidis N. MHC, TSP, and the origin of species: From immunogenetics to evolutionary genetics. Annual Review of Genetics. 2007;**41**:281-304

[9] Garrigan D, Hedrick PW. Perspective: Detecting adaptive molecular polymorphism: Lessons from the MHC. Evolution. 2003;**57**(8):1707-1722

[10] Edwards SV, Hedrick PW. Evolution and ecology of MHC molecules: From genomics to sexual selection. Trends in Ecology & Evolution. 1998;**13**(8):305-311

[11] Sommer S. The importance of immune gene variability (MHC) in evolutionary ecology and conservation. Frontiers in Zoology. 2005;**2**(1):16

[12] Piertney SB, Oliver MK. The evolutionary ecology of the major histocompatibility complex. Heredity. 2006;**96**(1):7

[13] Bontadini A. HLA techniques: Typing and antibody detection in the laboratory of immunogenetics. Methods. 2012;**56**(4):471-476

[14] Cano P et al. Common and well-documented HLA alleles: Report of the ad-hoc Committee of the American Society for Histocompatibility and Immunogenetics. Human Immunology. 2007;**68**(5):392-417

[15] Messemaker TC, Huizinga TW, Kurreeman F. Immunogenetics of rheumatoid arthritis: Understanding functional implications. Journal of Autoimmunity. 2015;**64**:74-81

Chapter 2

Dynamic Interaction between Immune Escape Mechanism and HLA-Ib Regulation

*Gia-Gia Toni Ho, Funmilola Heinen, Florian Stieglitz,
Rainer Blasczyk and Christina Bade-Döding*

Abstract

HLA molecules scan the intracellular proteome and present self- or non-self-peptides to immune effector cells. HLA-Ia (HLA-A, HLA-B and HLA-C) are the most polymorphic genes, resulting in various numbers of allelic variants expressed on the surface of almost all nucleated cells. In contrast to HLA-Ia molecules that activate the immune system during pathogenic invasion, the marginal polymorphic HLA-Ib molecules (HLA-E, HLA-F and HLA-G) are upregulated during pathogenic episodes and mediate immune tolerance. A fine tuning between downregulation of HLA-Ia and upregulation of HLA-Ib can be observed through immunological episodes that require to remain unrecognized by immune effector cells. While HLA-Ia molecules collaborate by presenting a wide range of peptides, every HLA-Ib molecule is highly specialized in its protective immune function and seems to be restricted in the presentation of peptides. Additionally, Ia molecules are expressed ubiquitously while the expression of HLA-Ib molecules is strictly restricted to certain tissues and occurs instantly on demand of the cells/tissue that attempt to be hidden from the immune system. The more knowledge becomes available for the function of HLA-Ib molecules; the question emerges if the molecular typing of HLA-Ib molecules would be reasonable to take a decision post treatment for personalized cellular therapies.

Keywords: HLA-Ia, HLA-Ib, immune modulation, immune escape

1. Introduction

Human leukocyte antigens (HLA) are responsible for the regulation of the immune system. HLA molecules scan the proteome and present self- or non-self-peptides to immune effector cells [1]. T cells are highly specific and genetically restricted to recognizing HLA molecules. The capability of immune effector cells to recognize HLA-bound peptides is called MHC restriction and was first discovered by Zinkernagel and Doherty [2]. During pathogenic episodes, e.g. viral infection, the interaction between peptide and HLA-Ia (HLA-A, HLA-B and HLA-C) molecules with T cell receptors activates the immune system and enables the surveillance of the health statues of the cell. HLA molecules present an abundance of peptide antigens to T cells for a continuous immune surveillance through different infectious/pathogenic stages. Peptides are bound by certain amino acids (AAs) located in the α1 and/or α3 domain of the HLA heavy chain (hc), those AAs form a cleft, the peptide-binding region (PBR). Alterations in the PBR are crucial to achieve maximum diversity of the selectable and presentable antigen repertoire [3, 4]. Consequently, HLA-Ia molecules are the most polymorphic genes in the human genome, resulting in various numbers of allelic variants expressed on the surface of almost all nucleated cells [1].

Furthermore, the human genome contains HLA-Ib genes like HLA-E, HLA-F and HLA-G. Contrary to HLA-Ia molecules, they exhibit only a few polymorphisms [5]. HLA-Ib molecules differ not only in their limited polymorphisms from HLA-Ia molecules but also in their restricted peptide repertoire and their distinct tissue distribution [6–8]. Typically, the function of classical HLA-Ia molecules is the presentation of peptide antigens to immune effector cells, yet HLA-Ib molecules exhibit a diverse range of functions in innate and adaptive immunity. In recent years, HLA-Ib molecules play a fundamental role in the understanding of virus-induced immunopathology, pathogen recognition, tumor immunosurveillance and regulation of autoimmunity [9–11]. In contrast to HLA-Ia molecules that activate the immune system during pathogenic invasion, the marginal polymorphic HLA-Ib molecules are upregulated during pathogenic episodes and mediate immune tolerance. A fine tuning between the downregulation of HLA-Ia molecules and the individual upregulation of highly specialized HLA-Ib molecules can be observed through immunological episodes that require to remain unrecognized by immune effector cells [12–14].

HLA-E features a specialized role between HLA and the immune system through engagement between innate and adaptive immunity; its interaction with an NK cell receptor or the T cell receptor could be distinguished [6, 15, 16]. During viral infections, viral immune evasion proteins disable through distinct actions: (i) the loading of peptides on HLA molecules, (ii) the trafficking of peptide-loaded HLA molecules to the cell surface or (iii) the retention of imma-ture or mature peptide-HLA complexes in the endoplasmic reticulum. These entire virus-mediated actions result in infected cells that do not present peptide-HLA complexes on their surface and would be susceptible to NK cell-mediated lysis. HLA-E is upregulated in infected cells during infection and protects infected HLA-Ia empty cells from being recognized by NK cells [17, 18]. HLA-G is only expressed in restricted tissue, exclusively in immune-privileged sites. The protec-tive potential of HLA-G is expressed through the capability of HLA-G to alter the phenotype of cytotoxic T cells towards non-reactive Tregs. HLA-G is the ligand for different NK cell receptors dependent on the tissue where it is expressed. Additionally, HLA-G can be found as membrane bound and soluble isoforms. In comparison to the other Ib molecules, HLA-G exhibits a unique molecular structure and diverse modulatory function in immune response [19, 20]. The presence of HLA-G is associated with immune tolerance. It is expressed in immune-privileged tissues, e.g. cornea and placenta [21]. It confers protection to the fetus from destruction by the maternal immune system during pregnancy and displays an immune checkpoint molecule in tumor immune evasion strategies [22, 23]. Among the Ib molecules, HLA-F is still an enigma. It is known that HLA-F molecule is a ligand for KIR3DS1 receptor on NK cells [24]. One remarkable immune function is its upregulation on the surface of HIV-infected CD4$^+$ T cells [25] where it enables NK cells to recognize the infection and destroy the infected host cells.

The aim of this chapter is to focus on the role of HLA-Ib during pathogenic episodes and their position in immunomodulatory mechanisms.

2. HLA-E

The *HLA-E* gene is located on the short arm of chromosome 6 and is composed of eight exons. In contrast to the other HLA-Ib molecules, HLA-E shows a broad tissue distribution. HLA-E is expressed in all nucleated cells [26]. Among the HLA molecules HLA-E is the least polymorphic; and proteins only 27 allelic variants enoding for 8 proteins are known [27]. However, of the described coding HLA-E variants, only two functional variants HLA-E*01:01 and HLA-E*01:03 are predomi-nately distributed in the population. The frequency of both allelic variants in the population is approximately equal [28]. HLA-E*01:01 and HLA-E*01:03 differ only in one amino acid (AA) substitution at position 107 located in the α2 domain. An arginine for HLA-E*01:01 is substituted by a glycine for HLA-E*01:03. Interestingly, this polymorphism in contrast to the classical HLA molecules is not located in the PBR. A substitution at this position is unlikely influencing peptide presentation. We recently, however, demonstrated that this single polymorphism affects its immune function considerably [14]. Peptide studies utilizing soluble HLA technology revealed a shift in the peptide-binding repertoire between these two alleles [13, 29]. Despite the availability of the same proteomic content, HLA-E*01:03 selected and presented a smaller set of peptides than E*01:01; moreover, the C-terminal peptide-binding motif was altered towards a preference for lysine [13]. In comparison to HLA-E*01:01, the allelic variant HLA-E*01:03 shows higher thermal stability and higher level of surface expression [5]. Furthermore, clinical studies that analyzed the role of HLA-E allelic subtypes in hematopoietic stem cell transplantation (HSCT) showed the clinical relevance of HLA-E matching and recommended prospective HLA-E screening pre-HSCT. The analysis of the overall survival, non-relapse mortality and disease-free survival revealed that HLA-E incompatibility however significantly improves these factors [30].

Like classical HLA-Ia molecules, HLA-E forms a trimeric complex consisting of the heavy chain, β2-microglobuline (β2m) and a peptide (pHLA) that is presented on the cell surface [31]. The main protein source of HLA-E-restricted peptides is the leader sequence derived from other HLA molecules. Thus, the expression level of other HLA molecules determines the surface expression of HLA-E. Peptide binding studies with random peptide libraries show that HLA-E is also capable of binding peptides from stress signals or pathogens [32]. The peptide-binding features of HLA-E indicate its special immunomodulatory qualities. Due to the low polymorphism of HLA-E, the fine tuning of HLA-E immune response is exclusively dependent on the bound antigenic peptide.

2.1 Immunomodulatory qualities of HLA-E

HLA-E exhibits a dual role in the immune system. On the one hand, HLA-E regulates the innate immunity through interaction with the NK cell receptor, and on the other hand, it can activate the adaptive immunity through interaction with the T cell receptor. The interaction of HLA-E with the respective immune effector cell depends considerably on the peptide presented on HLA-E (**Figure 1**) [6, 15, 16].

HLA-E is a mediator of NK cell inhibition and activation. HLA-E constitutes a ligand for both the inhibitory CD94/NKG2A and the stimulatory CD94/NKG2C NK cell receptor on NK cells. The reason for the differential binding to these functionally diverse receptors could be explained by the presentation of a diverse set of peptides. We could demonstrate an unknown HLA-E peptide-driven NK cell reactivity [14]. Through surface plasmon resonance (SPR) binding studies where the same peptide sequence derived from leader peptides of HLA-Ia molecules have been used to assemble pHLA-E complexes, it could be demonstrated that the HLA-E-binding affinity differs between these two NKG2 subunits. HLA-E binds CD94/NKG2A with a higher affinity than CD94/NKG2C [33]. The main peptide source of HLA-E is the leader sequence of HLA-Ia molecules; therefore, the role of HLA-E in innate immunity is to present HLA-E bound to these peptides to NK cells to inhibit NK-mediated lysis through pHLA-E/CD94/NKG2A engagement [7].

In adaptive immunity, certain HLA-E peptide complexes can be recognized by CD8+ T cells [34]. In addition to the presentation of self-peptides, HLA-E can also present a various number of pathogen-derived peptides, and these pHLA-E complexes elicit specific T cell responses. Although peptides presented by HLA-E are very restricted, it could be demonstrated that peptides derived from Epstein-Barr virus (EBV) [35], Cytomegalovirus (CMV) [36] or hepatitis C virus (HCV) [37] can be presented by HLA-E and recognized by virus-specific T cells. Furthermore, it has been reported that HLA-E also binds bacteria-derived peptides from Mycobacterium tuberculosis (Mtb) [38] and Salmonella enterica serovar Typhi [39]. These bacteria-derived peptides do not prevent NK-mediated lysis; instead, they elicit CD8+ T cell response [40, 41]. Like HLA-Ia-activated T cells, they combat intracellular bacteria through lysis of infected target cells [41]. However, interestingly, the HLA-E-specific CD8+ T cells uniquely produce Th2 (Il-4, Il-5, IL-13) cytokines instead of Th1 cytokines. Through B cell activation assays, it could be demonstrated that the T cells activate B cells that are able to induce cytokine production (**Figure 1**; [41]). These findings emphasize the important role of HLA-E in the adaptive immune response. It becomes obvious that also viruses and tumor cells use HLA-E for their own advantage to escape T cell recognition.

2.2 HLA-E in tumors

In order to evade CTL recognition due to tumor-peptide presentation, the downregulation of HLA molecules is a widespread mechanism of tumor cells.

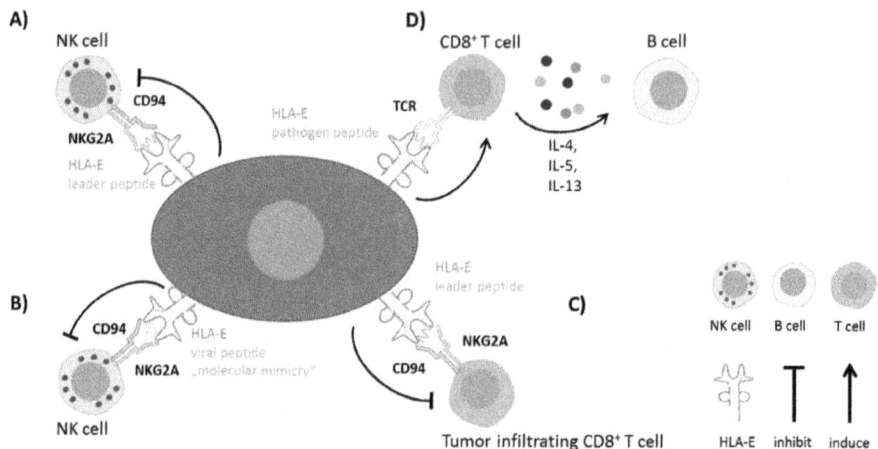

Figure 1.
The multiple roles of HLA-E in immune system. (A) HLA-E presents leader peptides to the unique inhibitory heterodimeric CD94/NKG2A receptor present on NK cells. (B) As part of immune evasion, HCMV glycoprotein UL40 provides a peptide mimicking the leader sequence of HLA-Ia molecules, thus inhibiting the NK cell by providing a ligand for CD94/NKG2A receptor. (C) As part of tumor immune evasion, the expression of the inhibitory NK cell receptor CD94/NKG2A is upregulated on tumor infiltrating CD8+ T cell leading to an inhibitory effect on these cells. (D) HLA-E can bind pathogenic peptides and elicit a CD8+ T cell response. Through HLA-E binding, CD8+ T cells release Th2 cytokines (IL-4, IL-5 and IL-13) and activate B cells.

Interestingly, the expression of HLA-E and HLA-G is upregulated in various types of cancers [42], indicating the use of these molecules as a special mechanism for immune evasion [9]. The cellular surface expression of pHLA complexes is required to avoid NK cell-mediated lysis. During tumor escape episodes, pHLA-Ia expression is downregulated; however, the expression of the HLA hc remains mostly unaffected, enabling the assembly of HLA-Ia hc and HLA-E. Since those pHLA-E complexes inhibit the NK cell reaction through its interaction with CD94/NKG2A, HLA-E expression provides an advantage for survival of the tumor cell. Furthermore, novel insights from cancer research suggest that the expression of HLA-E contributes to disease progression and is associated with a poor clinical prognosis [43, 44]. In patient with cervical and ovarian cancer, tumor infiltrating CD8$^+$ CTLs showed a higher expression of the CD94/NKG2A inhibitory receptor, and only a very low number of NK cells were found in tumor tissues (**Figure 1**) [45–47]. Regarding to the high expression of HLA-E in these tissues, those findings lead to the assumption that HLA-E plays a protective role and benefits the tumor through inhibition of CD94$^+$/NKG2A$^+$ CTLs and recognition of NK cells. Additionally, immunohistochemically stained breast cancer tissues showed that HLA-E expression is a prognostic marker for tumor progression [48]. Also in patients with non-small cell lung cancer (NSCLC), immunohistochemical staining demonstrated the association of HLA-E expression with a worse outcome for survival especially in the cells that are HLA-Ia negative and HLA-E positive [49]. In studies on colorectal cancer, an overexpression of HLA-E correlated with the malignancy stage. Remarkably, the release of soluble HLA-E could be detected in these cells [50]. In recent years, the focus of soluble HLA-Ib molecules as potential biomarker increased. In particular, soluble HLA-E and HLA-G are in the focus, because their expression is highly associated with the disease progression in tumor cells. In case of HLA-E, soluble molecules were significantly increased in neuroblastoma [51], melanoma [52] and chronic lymphocytic leukemia [53]. However, the overexpression of HLA-E is associated with the inhibition of tumor infiltrating NK cells and CD94$^+$/NKG2A$^+$ CTLs and contributes as one factor for the immune evasion strategies of tumor cells.

2.3 HLA-E in viral infections

Downregulation of HLA-Ia molecules is not only an escape mechanism of tumor cells but also a mechanism of pathogens like viruses. Human cytomegalovirus (HCMV) is one of the most intensive investigated pathogen related to HLA immune evasion. HCMV encodes several proteins that interfere with the antigen presentation and HLA expression. The glycoproteins US2 and US11 redirect the HLA hc from endoplasmic reticulum (ER) to the cytosol and induce the proteasomal degradation of the molecule. US3 inhibits the tapasin-dependent peptide loading leading to the retention of the HLA hc in the ER. Glycoprotein US6 inhibits the function of TAP. The loss of ligands for the inhibitory receptor increased the risk of NK cell recognition of the infected cells and for that reason HCMV developed mechanisms that inhibit NK cell responses [54]. One of these mechanisms involves the expression of HLA-E. HCMV encodes for the glycoprotein UL40. This protein has the same nonapeptide sequence (VMAPRTLIL) as the leader sequence of different HLA-C alleles that can bind to HLA-E [17] and thus inhibit NK cell-mediated lysis. TAP is a protein from the peptide loading complex (PLC) that is fundamental for the loading of peptides into the HLA PBR. TAP deficiency results in the presentation of empty HLA molecules on the cell surface. Interestingly, HLA-E expression analysis in TAP-deficient cells showed that HLA-E binds the HCMV peptide TAP-independently [17, 55]. Thus, UL40 can inhibit the NK cell recognition via HLA-E, even when the other HCMV glycoproteins prevent the presentation of pHLA-Ia complexes. HCMV utilizes the protective effect of HLA-E towards NK cell lysis through molecular mimicry (**Figure 1**). Furthermore, it could be demonstrated that UL40 polymorphism in HCMV impacts the recognition of HLA-E by NK cells. SPR analysis and cytotoxicity assays with 14 UL40 polymorphisms were performed to confirm that the binding affinity of HLA-E and CD94/NKG2A or CD94/NKG2C and the mediated reaction depend on the presented peptide [56]. These studies show that the alteration of the peptide sequence influences the recognition by CD94/NKG2A or CD94/NKG2C significantly and consequently impacts NK cell-mediated cytotoxicity. The HCV protein YLLPRRGPRL also binds into the PBR of HLA-E. Thus, peptides of other viruses also stabilized the HLA-E expression on infected cells and reduced the NK cell-mediated toxicity [57]. These findings show that the peptide presentation on HLA-E impairs the interaction with NK cell receptors considerably.

3. HLA-G

Among the very oligomorphic family of HLA-Ib molecules, HLA-G is the most polymorphic representative with 58 different alleles compared to 27 and 30 alleles of HLA-E and HLA-F, respectively [27]. The *HLA-G* gene is located on chromosome 6p21.3 close to HLA-A locus and is composed of eight exons with an internal stop codon after Exon 6. Through intron variability, those 58 encode eventually for 17 proteins. HLA-G*01:01 resembles the most common variant worldwide; in Europe, it is followed by HLA-G*01:04 and HLA-G*01:03 [58]. Mediated by alternative splicing, four membrane-bound (HLA-G1-G4) and three (HLA-G5-G7) soluble isoforms of HLA-G exist [59, 60]. The full-length membrane bound molecule is resembled by the HLA-G1 isoform, and its soluble equivalents are either generated by a stop codon after Exon 4 (HLA-G5) or by cleaving the membrane bound HLA-G1 from cell surface (soluble HLA-G1). The cleaving process of HLA-G1 is mediated by IL-10-dependent matrix metalloproteinase-2 (MMP2) [61]. The cleaving process was verified through coincubation of MMP2 with HLA-G-expressing cells and IL-10. A sharp increase in soluble HLA-G1 could be detected, whereas HLA-G5 mRNA levels remain constant [61]. MMP2 is predominantly expressed in the placenta and the lung [6]. The other membrane-bound isoforms are generated through elimination of one or more α-domains and for the soluble equivalents a stop codon after Exon 4 or Exon 2 (HLA-G7) (**Figure 2**). So far, receptors are reported only for the isoforms HLA-G2 and HLA-G6 [62]. The most expressed isoforms appear to be HLA-G1 and HLA-G5 [63–65]. For the membrane-bound isoforms (HLA-G2–HLA-G4), it could be shown that they could be detected on cell surface of transfected cells [66], whereas for the soluble isoforms only HLA-G5 and HLA-G6 (only after transplantation [67]) could be detected in supernatant of transfected cells as well as in the blood [65]. Nevertheless, it could be demonstrated that the membrane-bound isoforms convey also a protective status as well as HLA-G1 despite their different α-domain composition [33]. In addition, a recent study could demonstrate that HLA-G2 and HLA-G6 could bind to ILT4 through their α3 domain [62] but not to ILT2 due to the fact that the ILT2 binding to HLA-G is β2m-dependent [68]. Those findings suggest that the biological function and implementation of HLA-G are crucially depending on its structure. Nevertheless, despite those findings, it is not known yet whether the isoforms of HLA-G1 and HLA-G5 are relevant *in vivo* under physiological conditions [62].

In terms of peptide presentation, HLA-G differs from other HLA-Ib molecules like HLA-E that presents a very restricted peptide repertoire derived from the signal sequence of other HLA molecules irrespectively of the HLA-E-expressing tissue [7]. In contrast, HLA-G is considered to be a classical peptide presenter like HLA-Ia molecules; however, its peptide repertoire is restricted to the tissue distribution and cell type [7, 69, 70]. Peptide identification of HLA subtypes is usually performed by affinity purification of the desired HLA molecule from a selected tissue/cell type followed by peptide isolation and mass spectrometric sequencing. A reason for the detection of a restricted HLA-G peptide repertoire might therefore be the selection of the HLA-G-expressing tissue/cell type or the unintended selection of HLA-G*01:01 exclusively. We recently demonstrated that the HLA-G-restricted peptide repertoire is distinctively determined by the HLA-G allelic subtype. Despite the fact that the allelic variants HLA-G*01:04, HLA-G*01:03 and HLA-G*01:01 differ from each other by a single AA in an outer loop position outside the PBR, the selected peptide repertoire and the peptide binding motif are fundamentally different [12].

While the HLA-Ib molecule HLA-E and HLA-Ia molecules are ubiquitously expressed on every nucleated cell, HLA-G expression is restricted under physiological conditions to immune privileged sites. HLA-G is expressed in placenta [71], thymus [72], cornea [21], nail matrix [73], pancreas [74] and erythroid and endothelial precursors [75]. Also, HLA-G is ectopically expressed in transplanted organs, tumors, monocytes, viral infections and autoimmune diseases [76–78].

3.1 HLA-G in pregnancy

Under healthy conditions, the main expressing site of HLA-G is the placenta [79]. In the placenta, extravillous cytotrophoblast (EVT) cells are the only cells expressing membrane-bound HLA-G (G1) and secreting soluble HLA-G (G5) [79, 80]. The fetus can be considered a semi-allograft; hence the immune system of the mother has to be regulated in tolerogenic direction to avoid rejection. Here, HLA-G

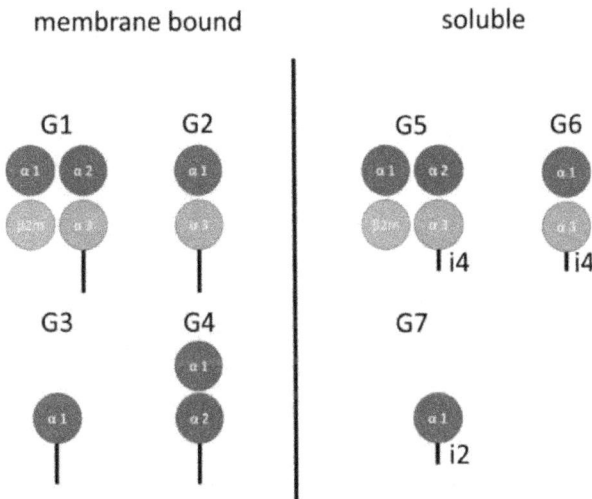

Figure 2.
Structural isoforms of HLA-G. Generation of HLA-G isoforms is done by alternative splicing of the HLA-G mRNA. HLA-G1 resembles the full-length membrane-bound HLA-G molecule. Membrane-bound isoforms are generated by abundance of certain α domains. Soluble isoforms are achieved by a stop codon after Exon 4 and Exon 2, respectively. Modified after Foroni et al. [7].

is the key element for maternal-fetal tolerance induction [80–82]. Interaction with HLA-G leads commonly to an inhibition of the interacting immune effector cells [83–86]. Those interactions are mediated through inhibiting receptors like KIR2DL4 and ILT2 on NK cells [87], ILT2 on T cells, ILT4 on macrophages and ILT4/CD160 on dendritic cells [88]. The binding site for those receptors is suggested to be the alpha-3 domain of HLA-G (G1 or G5) [89]. KIR2DL4 and ILT2 interaction leads to inhibition of NK-mediated lysis [87]. Additionally, it has been reported that at the maternal interface decidual NK cells (a unique immunosuppressive and proangiogenic subset of NK cells [90]; dNK) are up-taking and internalizing HLA-G from the EVT cellular surface via trogocytosis mediated by a yet not clearly identified receptor [91]. Internalization of HLA-G is necessary for maintaining a low cytotoxicity and immunosuppressive status of dNK cells. It could be shown that the disappearance of internal HLA-G leads to cytokine production and an overall higher cytotoxicity of dNK cells, the functional background of this mechanism is still unclear and further research has to be performed [91, 92]. Although, it is assumed that KIR2DL4, through its highly intracellular occurrence, is involved in an intracellular cascade leading to this immunosuppressive status [91]. Moreover, alloproliferative response of CD4$^+$ T cells is inhibited by ILT2 interaction with HLA-G [93], and the population is driven to a suppressive and passive phenotype [94]. Furthermore, it is known that HLA-G5 induces in ILT4$^+$ dendritic cells (DCs) the production of the immunosuppressive cytokine IL-10 and an arrest of matura-tion [95, 96] as well as the induction of Tregs (CD4$^+$ CD25^{high}FOXP3$^+$) [97] and Tr1 cells by IL-10-producing dendritic cells [96, 98]. Moreover, through interaction with the ILT2 receptor on B cells, HLA-G inhibits proliferation, differentiation and antibody secretion [85]. In addition, HLA-G5 induces apoptosis of CD8$^+$ T cells and

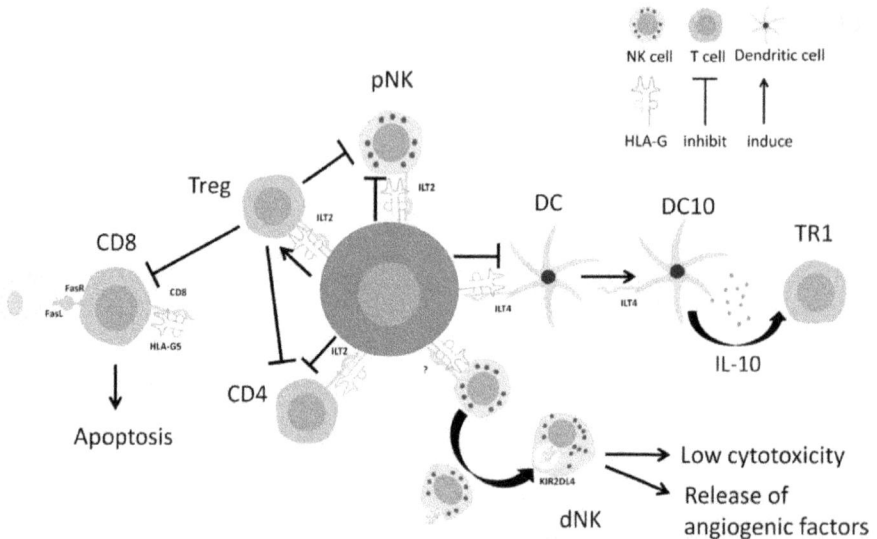

Figure 3.
HLA-G binding inhibiting immune effector cell activation. HLA-G regulates the immune system to an immunosuppressive and tolerogenic status by inducing the development of CD4$^+$ and CD8$^+$ to regulatory T cells and IL-10 production by DCs. Furthermore, HLA-G is able to inhibit CD4$^+$ and pNK cells directly through binding to ILT2. In addition, soluble HLA-G induces apoptosis in CD8$^+$ T cells by activation of the FasL/FasR pathway. Decidual NK cells are up-taking HLA-G from the extravillous cytotrophoblast cell surface by a yet unidentified receptor. Intracellular KIR2DL4 is assumed to be responsible for an intracellular cascade that leads to immunosuppressive status of decidual NK cells. Treg: T regulatory cell; pNK: peripheral natural killer cell; DC: dendritic cell; DC10: IL-10-producing dendritic cell; TR1: type 1 T regulatory cell; dNK: decidual natural killer cell; CD4: CD4$^+$ T cells; CD8: CD8$^+$ T cells. Modified after Rizzo et al. [78].

endothelial cells through interactions with CD8 receptor and activation of FasR/FasL pathway in CD8+ T cells and CD160 on endothelial cells (**Figure 3**) [69]. To conclude, HLA-G has a strong immunosuppressive impact and thus plays a critical role in maintaining an immunotolerant status in pregnancies.

3.2 Interactions of HLA-G

In recent years, the impact of the presented peptide on the interaction between HLA-G and its cognate receptors is controversially discussed. It has been reported that the interaction between HLA-G and its receptors is mediated exclusively by the HLA-G α3 domain and not by the α1 and/or α2 domain. Therefore, it was concluded that the presented peptide has no influence on the receptor-HLA-G interaction [68, 99], whereas we could demonstrate that the HLA-G alleles, HLA-G*01:01, G*01:03 and G*01:04, differing from each other by single AA polymorphism within the α2 region and a variability in peptide-binding features, convey a different degree in protection from NK cell-mediated lysis [12]. These results imply that the available membrane-bound HLA-G for a given NK cell receptor is influenced by the peptide-mediated alteration of the molecule [12]. Supporting our functional results, a recent study describes the x-ray structure of the D3D4 domain of the ILT2 receptor; this structural insight indicates that ILT2 would be theoretically able to interact with the α1 and α2 domain of an HLA-G molecule [100]. Taken all those findings into account, it seems apparent that the α3 domain is the main receptor-binding site of HLA-G; however, it should be considered that the α1 and α2 domain as well as the bound peptide directly or indirectly have a great impact on the HLA-G-NK-receptor interactions; therefore, it becomes obvious that the HLA-G allele has more functional impact than previously thought.

3.3 HLA-G in cancer

As a consequence of its immunosuppressive abilities, the ectopic expression of HLA-G1 is a part of immune evasion strategies of many tumors to escape immunosurveillance by T and NK lymphocytes [101]. In esophageal squamous cell carcinoma, heighten IL-10 and HLA-G levels could be detected and correlated with a poor outcome [102]. HLA-G was found to be an independent factor for overall survival in colorectal cancer [103]. Heighten soluble HLA-G levels were found in plasma levels of patients with chronic lymphatic leukemia, T-non-Hodgkin lymphoma (NHL), B-NHL [104], multiple myeloma [105] and breast cancer, whereas in the later one heighten soluble HLA-G levels are associated with a better outcome of neoadjuvant chemotherapy [19] In pancreatic cancer, HLA-G expression is common and positively correlated with metastasis and a worse overall survival [106]. In essence, HLA-G ectopic expression in tumors is common and correlated with tumor progression and patients' survival as recent studies could demonstrate [101].

3.4 HLA-G in transplantations

In past years, HLA-G has received more and more attention as a potential biomarker in transplantations due to its immunomodulatory abilities [107]. It could be shown that myocardial HLA-G expression is correlated with low risk of acute cellular rejection in heart transplant recipients [108]. In lung transplantation, acute rejections were observed in patients without HLA-G expression in the donor lung, whereas in stable patients, HLA-G expression was frequently detected. Also, in long-term follow-ups, HLA-G expression correlated significantly with a lower occurrence of steroid-resistant acute rejection and bronchiolitis obliterans syndrome [109]. Furthermore, HLA-G expression in biliary epithelial cells is positively correlated with an overall better acceptance in liver-kidney transplantations [110]. Moreover, it could be shown that HLA-G expression in endomyocardial biopsies is negatively correlated with C4d staining, a marker for antibody-mediated rejection, implying that HLA-G expression protects the graft from antibody-mediated rejection [111]. Contrastingly, heighten levels of membrane-bound isoforms (G1 and G3) combined with lower amount of G5 corresponded with acute rejection in end-stage renal disease [107, 112]. Although HLA-G seems to play a critical role in terms of graft acceptance and long-term survival, it is however not comprehensively used as a biomarker, yet.

Given the fact that HLA-G expression is often correlated with a better graft acceptance, LeMaoult et al. investigated HLA-G as a potential therapeutic target to improve graft acceptance. By utilizing synthetic HLA-G molecules, they could demonstrate that synthetic HLA-G molecules are capable of improving skin graft survival and tolerance induction in mice [113]. These findings underline the pivotal role of HLA-G for transplantations in the future.

3.5 HLA-G in autoimmune diseases and inflammation

In the context of autoimmune and inflammatory diseases, several studies have investigated the role of HLA-G that controls the disease progression [101]. In return, HLA-G polymorphisms and expression levels have been linked to several autoimmune/inflammatory diseases such as ulcerative colitis (UC) [78], Crohn's disease [101], celiac disease [114], psoriasis [115], pemphigus vulgaris [116], rheumatoid arthritis [117] and multiple sclerosis [78, 101]. Ulcerative colitis and Crohn's disease are both inflammatory gastrointestinal diseases in which sHLA-G secretion by peripheral blood mononuclear cells (PBMCs) could serve as a marker to distinguish between them and further could be utilized for controlling treatment progression [118]. PBMCs from healthy patient and patients with UC do not secrete sHLA-G under physiological conditions, whereas PBMCs from patients with Crohn's disease secrete sHLA-G. This pathological pattern reverses under immunosuppressive treatment PBMCs from UC patients start secreting sHLA-G whereas secretion is reduced in Crohn's disease patients [78, 119]. In chronic skin inflammation such as pemphigus vulgaris, heighten HLA-G expression could be observed [120] together with a higher frequency of HLA-G 14 bp DEL allele [116]. These findings advocate the role of HLA-G expression as a pivotal determinant in the evolution of pemphigus vulgaris [101]. In multiple sclerosis (MS), several studies indicate that HLA-G downregulates the autoinflammatory reaction in the microenvironment of the brain, and it could be shown that HLA-G suppresses cytokine production and CD4$^+$ T cell proliferation of MS patients *in vitro*. In addition, it has been found that sHLA-G serum levels are heighten *post-partum* in patients without clinical attacks [121], and a suppressive subset of CD4$^+$CD8$^+$ HLA-G secreting and expressing regulatory T cells could be observed in MS patients [122–124]. Contrastingly, a recent correlation analysis could find no significant evidence for an impact of sHLA-G levels on any parameter of multiple sclerosis [125].

3.6 HLA-G in infection diseases

Infection diseases can be divided into three groups (bacterial, parasitic and viral infection) in which HLA-G is associated with different outcomes and different diseases progression [126].

3.7 HLA-G in bacterial infections

As consequence of a far advanced bacterial infection, a septic shock leads to a systemic inflammation and is defined by a high fatality rate [127]. In this scenario, a highly increased HLA-G5 expression is correlated with a higher chance for survival by supporting the anti-inflammatory feedback loop [127].

3.8 HLA-G in parasitic infections

Toxoplasma gondii infection leads often to adverse pregnancy outcomes such as miscarriage and still birth [128]. It has been shown that *Toxoplasma gondii infection* leads to a higher secretion of sHLA-G by extravillous cytotrophoblast. Notably, those heightened sHLA-G expression leads to apoptosis of dNK cells when they were co-cultured with *Toxoplasma gondii*-infected extravillous cytotrophoblast [101]. Contrastingly, in healthy pregnancies, sHLA-G is a necessary factor for dNK cells to maintain their immunosuppressive and cytokine production status in order to sustain a correct placentation [91]. In conclusion, this differing mechanism could be one key determinant for a poor outcome of pregnancies while *Toxoplasma gondii infection.*

A recent study has observed a correlation of high maternal HLA-G serum levels with low birth weight and a higher risk of *Plasmodium falciparum* infection in infancy. Suggesting sHLA-G levels could be utilized as biomarker for sensitivity of infants for malaria infection [129].

3.9 HLA-G in viral infections

Commonly, sHLA-G levels are uprising during viral infection such as infections with HIV, hCMV, HCV and HBV [126]. This is due to heightened levels of cytokine production especially due to interferon secretion that stimulates HLA-G shedding from cell surface mediated by metalloproteases during viral infection [126]. During viral infection, IL-10 serum levels rise to dampening the proinflammatory TH1 immune response [130]. As a consequence, the IL-10-dependent MMP2 is activated and cleaved HLA-G1 from cell surface; this leads to a rise in soluble HLA-G1 levels [61].

In hCMV, increased membrane bound and soluble HLA-G levels could be detected during infection. It could also be shown that macrophages derived from latency infected monocytes upregulating HLA-G expression when the hCMV infection reactivates in order to avoid recognition by the immune system [131]. Further, sHLA-G serum level correlates with IL-10 and IFN-γ concentration due to IL-10- and interferon-dependent MMP [126].

In HBV and HCV infections, HLA-G serum levels also correlate with IL-10 and IFN-γ concentration. Furthermore, sHLA-G levels were observed to be higher in the chronic HBV situation than in the acute infection. In addition, higher HLA-G expression has been correlated with fibrotic areas within the liver in patients with a chronic HCV infection [132–135].

In context of HLA-G and viral infections, HIV infection is currently the most widely researched [126]. In HIV infections, HLA-G is expressed on nearly all monocytes and on 34% of T-cells [136]. HLA-G serum levels increased during first phase of infection and lowered to normal again when infection progresses to a chronic stage [136, 137]. If HLA-G serum levels remain high during infection progression, it indicates a fast progressor [136]. On basis of this change in HLA-G serum levels, it is proposed that HLA-G can be utilized as a biomarker for disease progression [126]. In addition, under antiretroviral therapy, serum

HLA-G levels decreased significantly and are correlated with virus clearance and an increase of CD4[+] T lymphocytes [126]. This is probably due to a decrease of an immune response and decreasing IL-10 and interferon levels. Furthermore, it is suggested that HLA-G-expressing monocytes serve as reservoir in HIV-infected patients, since they are protected from an immune response through their HLA-G surface expression [136]. In coherency to those findings, it is reported that HLA-G null allele, HLA-G*01:05 N allele, correlates with a lower risk of a HIV infection, whereas HLA-G*01:01:08 correlates with a higher risk of getting a HIV infection [138, 139]. Null alleles are characterized by a mutation that leads to a non-functional molecule [140]. Consequently, in patients with the allelic variant HLA-G*01:05 N, monocytes could not be served as HIV reservoir in an infection, because they are no longer protected from the immune system by a functional HLA-G expression [126].

4. HLA-F

The *HLA-F* gene is located on chromosome 6p21.3 telomeric to the HLA-A locus and is composed of seven exons. Exon 6 contains an internal stop codon leading to the exclusion of Exon 7 from the mature mRNA transcript. The association of HLA-F hc with β2m forms a 40–41 kDa protein with a truncated cytoplasmic tail [141, 142]. It has been proposed that this distinct cytoplasmic tail enables HLA-F to conquer the cell surface independent of the classical peptide-loading pathway in the ER [143].

Like HLA-E and HLA-G, HLA-F has limited allelic polymorphism when compared to the allelic variances of HLA-Ia molecules. Until now, 30 alleles encoding for five proteins (HLA-F*01:01, F*01:02, F*01:03, F*01:04, F*01:05) have been described [27].

AA residues within the PBR of HLA class I molecules determine their biophysical properties and thereby the feature of bound peptides. Ten of these amino acid residues are highly conserved in all HLA class I PBRs, except HLA-F that shows alterations in five of them, implying an unidentified immune function of HLA-F. Four of these alterations are located within the α1 domain where a methionine is substituted by a leucine at position 5, a tyrosine by a phenylalanine at position 22, a glycine by a glutamine at position 26 and a tyrosine by an arginine at position 84. The fifth alteration is located within the α1 domain with a substitution of phenylalanine for leucine at position 146 [141]. On this account, the electrostatic characteristics of the PBR are modified and HLA-F exclusive. It could be demonstrated that HLA-F-presented peptides are not restricted by length, because the A pocket of the PBR is blocked off due to the aforementioned substitutions. This allows binding of peptides of 7 to >30 AA in length that is more consistent with HLA class II molecules [144].

HLA-F expression is highly cell- and tissue-specific. Expression of HLA-F has been detected intracellularly in leukocytes, including monocytes, B cells, T cells and NK cells, as well as on the cell surface of activated lymphocytes excluding Treg cells [145]. As well as HLA-G and HLA-E, HLA-F has been detected on extravillous trophoblasts invading maternal decidua [146], even though its function during pregnancy is still unclear. It has been found that HLA-F underexpression due to single nucleotide polymorphisms (SNP) within the *HLA-F* gene correlates with reduced fecundity [147], suggesting a role in maternal-fetal tolerance.

In contrast to other HLA class I molecules, HLA-F has been described to be expressed as an open conformer (OC) without association with β2m and peptides; however, the usual trimeric hc/β2 m/peptide complexes could be detected as well.

These distinct HLA-F conformers are recognized by various binding partners of the NK cell receptor (NKR) family. While HLA-F OCs are mainly recognized by the killer cell immunoglobulin-like NKRs (KIR) KIR3DL2, KIR3DS4 [148] and KIR3DS1 [25], peptide-bound HLA-F complexes are ligands for the NKRs of the leukocyte immunoglobulin-like receptor (LIR) family, ILT2 and ILT4 [8, 144].

4.1 HLA-F in viral infections

HLA-F is the most enigmatic HLA-Ib molecule and little is known about its function. It has been found that through interaction with the KIR3DS1 receptor, HLA-F has a beneficial effect on HIV outcome.

Stimulation of KIR3DS1$^+$ and KIR3DS1$^-$ NK cell lines (NKCLs) with recombinant HLA-F monomers elicits downstream immune responses as production of antiviral cytokines (IFNγ, TNFα and MIP1β) measured by intracellular staining and NK cell degranulation measured by surface expression of the lysosome-associated marker CD107a in KIR3DS1$^+$ NKCLS, but not in KIR3DS1$^-$ NKCLs. Moreover, *in vitro* studies showed that KIR3DS1$^+$ NKCLs reduce the quantitative frequency of HIV-infected cells elucidating that KIR3DS1-HLA-F ligation inhibits HIV-1 replication (**Figure 4**). Interestingly, *HLA-F* transcription is upregulated in HIV-1-infected activated CD4$^+$ T cells. However, recognition of HLA-F by KIR3DS1 is weakened in 'early' infected cells that are characterized by low HIV p24 expression, CD4 positivity and HLA-Ia and tetherin expression and particularly diminished in 'late' infected cells with high p24 expression, low CD4 positivity and low HLA-Ia and tetherin expression, implying the involvement of HLA-F in an immune evasion strategy of HIV-1 [25].

4.2 HLA-F in tumors

Tumor cells evolved strategies to evade the immune system. One of the most frequently used mechanisms is the alteration of HLA expression, including the downregulation of HLA-Ia molecules to escape from recognition by cytotoxic T cells. HLA-Ib molecules exhibit protective features that protect the cells from NK cell lysis, and based on this, tumor cells upregulate these molecules for their own advantage.

In contrast to HLA-E and HLA-G, little is known about the function of HLA-F in tumor. Until now, HLA-F has been detected immunohistochemically in various cancers, i.e. non-small cell lung cancer (NSCLC) [149], esophageal squamous cell carcinoma [150], gastric adenocarcinoma [151] and breast cancer [152].

It has been reported that HLA-F detection is associated with a poor outcome in NSCLC and gastric adenocarcinoma. In patients with gastric adenocarcinoma, HLA-F detection leads to a more invasive carcinoma type and further lymph knot involvement and infiltration into blood vessels [151]. HLA-F has been found to

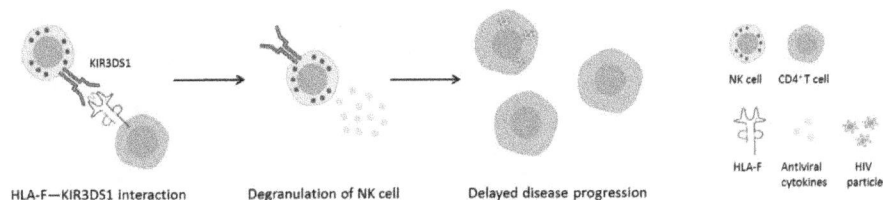

KIR3DS1

HLA-F—KIR3DS1 interaction   Degranulation of NK cell   Delayed disease progression

NK cell   CD4$^+$ T cell

HLA-F   Antiviral cytokines   HIV particle

Figure 4.
Effect of HLA-F-KIR3DS1 interaction on AIDS disease progression.

interact with the inhibitory NKRs, ILT2 and ILT4 [8], indicating its expression on tumor cells as protection against anticancer responses by the immune system. Yet in NSCLC, positive HLA-F expression is not associated with disease progression and differentiation status of the tumor [149]. The occurrence of HLA-F in breast cancer correlates with the size of tumor, but there is no evidence for nodal involvement [152].

Taken together, these findings imply organ-specific effects of HLA-F-positive tumors. Further investigation is necessary to verify and decode the underlying mechanism of tumor evasion strategies by cancers.

The immunomodulatory potential of HLA-F subtypic variants is still unknown. For that reason, we developed a typing strategy for typing HLA-F in certain patients (Ho et al., manuscript in preparation). It seems that the function of HLA-F as well as that of the other HLA-Ib molecules is influenced by the AA composition of the heavy chain. A single AA mismatch seems to tip the immunological balance (Ho et al., manuscript in preparation).

Taken together, the previously assumed invariability of the HLA-Ib heavy chain has to be rethought, and HLA-Ib typing seems to support intelligent patient management protocols.

Author details

Gia-Gia Toni Ho, Funmilola Heinen, Florian Stieglitz, Rainer Blasczyk and
Christina Bade-Döding*
Institute for Transfusion Medicine, Hannover Medical School, Hannover, Germany

*Address all correspondence to: bade-doeding.christina@mh-hannover.de

IntechOpen

© 2018 The Author(s). Licensee IntechOpen. This chapter is distributed under the terms
of the Creative Commons Attribution License (http://creativecommons.org/licenses/
by/3.0), which permits unrestricted use, distribution, and reproduction in any medium,
provided the original work is properly cited. (cc) BY

References

[1] Klein J, Sato A. The HLA system. First of two parts. The New England Journal of Medicine. 2000;**343**(10):702-709

[2] Zinkernagel RM, Doherty PC. Restriction of in vitro T cell-mediated cytotoxicity in lymphocytic choriomeningitis within a syngeneic or semiallogeneic system. Nature. 1974;**248**(5450):701-702

[3] Bade-Doeding C et al. A single amino-acid polymorphism in pocket a of HLA-A*6602 alters the auxiliary anchors compared with HLA-A*6601 ligands. Immunogenetics. 2004;**56**(2):83-88

[4] Bjorkman PJ et al. Structure of the human class I histocompatibility antigen, HLA-A2. Nature. 1987;**329**(6139):506-512

[5] Strong RK et al. HLA-E allelic variants. Correlating differential expression, peptide affinities, crystal structures, and thermal stabilities. The Journal of Biological Chemistry. 2003;**278**(7):5082-5090

[6] Kraemer T, Blasczyk R, Bade-Doeding C. HLA-E: A novel player for histocompatibility. Journal of Immunology Research. 2014;**2014**:352160

[7] Foroni I et al. HLA-E, HLA-F and HLA-G — The Non-Classical Side of the MHC Cluster, HLA and Associated Important Diseases Yongzhi Xi. IntechOpen. March 19th 2014. DOI: 10.5772/57507. Available from: https://www.intechopen.com/books/hla-and-associated-important-diseases/hla-e-hla-f-and-hla-g-the-non-classical-side-of-the-mhc-cluster

[8] Lepin EJ et al. Functional characterization of HLA-F and binding of HLA-F tetramers to ILT2 and ILT4 receptors. European Journal of Immunology. 2000;**30**(12):3552-3561

[9] Kochan G et al. Role of non-classical MHC class I molecules in cancer immunosuppression. Oncoimmunology. 2013;**2**(11):e26491

[10] Rebmann V et al. HLA-G as a tolerogenic molecule in transplantation and pregnancy. Journal of Immunology Research. 2014;**2014**:297073

[11] Hofstetter AR et al. Diverse roles of non-diverse molecules: MHC class Ib molecules in host defense and control of autoimmunity. Current Opinion in Immunology. 2011;**23**(1):104-110

[12] Celik AA et al. HLA-G mediated immune regulation is impaired by a single amino acid exchange in the alpha 2 domain. Human Immunology. 2018;**79**(6):453-462

[13] Celik AA et al. The diversity of the HLA-E-restricted peptide repertoire explains the immunological impact of the Arg107Gly mismatch. Immunogenetics. 2016;**68**(1):29-41

[14] Kraemer T et al. HLA-E: Presentation of a broader peptide repertoire impacts the cellular immune response-implications on HSCT outcome. Stem Cells International. 2015;**2015**:346714

[15] Posch PE et al. HLA-E is the ligand for the natural killer cell CD94/NKG2 receptors. Journal of Biomedical Science. 1998;**5**(5):321-331

[16] Pietra G et al. HLA-E and HLA-E-bound peptides: Recognition by subsets of NK and T cells. Current Pharmaceutical Design. 2009;**15**(28):3336-3344

[17] Tomasec P et al. Surface expression of HLA-E, an inhibitor of natural

killer cells, enhanced by human cytomegalovirus gpUL40. Science. 2000;**287**(5455):1031

[18] Guzman-Fulgencio M et al. HLA-E variants are associated with sustained virological response in HIV/hepatitis C virus-coinfected patients on hepatitis C virus therapy. AIDS. 2013;**27**(8):1231-1238

[19] Konig L et al. The prognostic impact of soluble and vesicular HLA-G and its relationship to circulating tumor cells in neoadjuvant treated breast cancer patients. Human Immunology. 2016;**77**(9):791-799

[20] Rebmann V et al. Detection of soluble HLA-G molecules in plasma and amniotic fluid. Tissue Antigens. 1999;**53**(1):14-22

[21] Le Discorde M et al. Expression of HLA-G in human cornea, an immune-privileged tissue. Human Immunology. 2003;**64**(11):1039-1044

[22] McMaster MT et al. Human placental HLA-G expression is restricted to differentiated cytotrophoblasts. Journal of Immunology. 1995;**154**(8):3771-3778

[23] Polakova K, Russ G. Expression of the non-classical HLA-G antigen in tumor cell lines is extremely restricted. Neoplasma. 2000;**47**(6):342-348

[24] Burian A et al. HLA-F and MHC-I open conformers bind natural killer cell Ig-like receptor KIR3DS1. PLoS One. 2016;**11**(9):e0163297

[25] Garcia-Beltran WF et al. Open conformers of HLA-F are high-affinity ligands of the activating NK-cell receptor KIR3DS1. Nature Immunology. 2016;**17**(9):1067-1074

[26] Braud V, Jones EY, McMichael A. The human major histocompatibility complex class Ib molecule HLA-E binds signal sequence-derived peptides with primary anchor residues at positions 2 and 9. European Journal of Immunology. 1997;**27**(5):1164-1169

[27] Robinson J et al. The IPD and IMGT/HLA database: Allele variant databases. Nucleic Acids Research. 2015;**43**(Database issue):D423-D431

[28] Grimsley C, Ober C. Population genetic studies of HLA-E: Evidence for selection. Human Immunology. 1997;**52**(1):33-40

[29] Kunze-Schumacher H, Blasczyk R, Bade-Doeding C. Soluble HLA technology as a strategy to evaluate the impact of HLA mismatches. Journal of Immunology Research. 2014;**2014**:246171

[30] Tsamadou C et al. Human leukocyte antigen-E mismatch is associated with better hematopoietic stem cell transplantation outcome in acute leukemia patients. Haematologica. 2017;**102**(11):1947-1955

[31] Petrie EJ et al. CD94-NKG2A recognition of human leukocyte antigen (HLA)-E bound to an HLA class I leader sequence. The Journal of Experimental Medicine. 2008;**205**(3):725-735

[32] Stevens J et al. Peptide binding characteristics of the non-classical class Ib MHC molecule HLA-E assessed by a recombinant random peptide approach. BMC Immunology. 2001;**2**:5

[33] Kaiser BK et al. Interactions between NKG2x immunoreceptors and HLA-E ligands display overlapping affinities and thermodynamics. Journal of Immunology. 2005;**174**(5):2878-2884

[34] Pietra G et al. The analysis of the natural killer-like activity of human cytolytic T lymphocytes revealed HLA-E as a novel target for TCR alpha/beta-mediated recognition.

European Journal of Immunology. 2001;**31**(12):3687-3693

[35] Jorgensen PB et al. Epstein-Barr virus peptide presented by HLA-E is predominantly recognized by CD8(bright) cells in multiple sclerosis patients. PLoS One. 2012;**7**(9):e46120

[36] Pietra G et al. HLA-E-restricted recognition of cytomegalovirus-derived peptides by human CD8+ cytolytic T lymphocytes. Proceedings of the National Academy of Sciences of the United States of America. 2003;**100**(19):10896-10901

[37] Schulte D et al. The HLA-E(R)/HLA-E(R) genotype affects the natural course of hepatitis C virus (HCV) infection and is associated with HLA-E-restricted recognition of an HCV-derived peptide by interferon-gamma-secreting human CD8(+) T cells. The Journal of Infectious Diseases. 2009;**200**(9):1397-1401

[38] Heinzel AS et al. HLA-E-dependent presentation of Mtb-derived antigen to human CD8+ T cells. The Journal of Experimental Medicine. 2002;**196**(11):1473-1481

[39] Salerno-Goncalves R et al. Identification of a human HLA-E-restricted CD8+ T cell subset in volunteers immunized with salmonella enterica serovar Typhi strain Ty21a typhoid vaccine. Journal of Immunology. 2004;**173**(9):5852-5862

[40] Caccamo N et al. Human CD8 T lymphocytes recognize mycobacterium tuberculosis antigens presented by HLA-E during active tuberculosis and express type 2 cytokines. European Journal of Immunology. 2015;**45**(4):1069-1081

[41] van Meijgaarden KE et al. Human CD8+ T-cells recognizing peptides from mycobacterium tuberculosis (Mtb) presented by

HLA-E have an unorthodox Th2-like, multifunctional, Mtb inhibitory phenotype and represent a novel human T-cell subset. PLoS Pathogens. 2015;**11**(3):e1004671

[42] Marin R et al. Analysis of HLA-E expression in human tumors. Immunogenetics. 2003;**54**(11):767-775

[43] Bossard C et al. HLA-E/beta2 microglobulin overexpression in colorectal cancer is associated with recruitment of inhibitory immune cells and tumor progression. International Journal of Cancer. 2012;**131**(4):855-863

[44] Wolpert F et al. HLA-E contributes to an immune-inhibitory phenotype of glioblastoma stem-like cells. Journal of Neuroimmunology. 2012;**250**(1-2):27-34

[45] Gooden M et al. HLA-E expression by gynecological cancers restrains tumor-infiltrating CD8(+) T lymphocytes. Proceedings of the National Academy of Sciences of the United States of America. 2011;**108**(26):10656-10661

[46] Sheu BC et al. Integration of high-risk human papillomavirus DNA correlates with HLA genotype aberration and reduced HLA class I molecule expression in human cervical carcinoma. Clinical Immunology. 2005;**115**(3):295-301

[47] Sheu BC et al. Up-regulation of inhibitory natural killer receptors CD94/NKG2A with suppressed intracellular perforin expression of tumor-infiltrating CD8+ T lymphocytes in human cervical carcinoma. Cancer Research. 2005;**65**(7):2921-2929

[48] de Kruijf EM et al. HLA-E and HLA-G expression in classical HLA class I-negative tumors is of prognostic value for clinical outcome of early breast cancer patients. Journal of Immunology. 2010;**185**(12):7452-7459

[49] Talebian Yazdi M et al. The positive prognostic effect of stromal CD8+ tumor-infiltrating T cells is restrained by the expression of HLA-E in non-small cell lung carcinoma. Oncotarget. 2016;7(3):3477-3488

[50] Levy EM et al. Human leukocyte antigen-E protein is overexpressed in primary human colorectal cancer. International Journal of Oncology. 2008;32(3):633-641

[51] Morandi F et al. Plasma levels of soluble HLA-E and HLA-F at diagnosis may predict overall survival of neuroblastoma patients. BioMed Research International. 2013;2013:956878

[52] Allard M et al. Serum soluble HLA-E in melanoma: A new potential immune-related marker in cancer. PLoS One. 2011;6(6):e21118

[53] Wagner B et al. HLA-E allelic genotype correlates with HLA-E plasma levels and predicts early progression in chronic lymphocytic leukemia. Cancer. 2017;123(5):814-823

[54] Jackson SE, Mason GM, Wills MR. Human cytomegalovirus immunity and immune evasion. Virus Research. 2011;157(2):151-160

[55] Ulbrecht M et al. HCMV glycoprotein US6 mediated inhibition of TAP does not affect HLA-E dependent protection of K-562 cells from NK cell lysis. Human Immunology. 2003;64(2):231-237

[56] Heatley SL et al. Polymorphism in human cytomegalovirus UL40 impacts on recognition of human leukocyte antigen-E (HLA-E) by natural killer cells. The Journal of Biological Chemistry. 2013;288(12):8679-8690

[57] Nattermann J et al. The HLA-A2 restricted T cell epitope HCV core 35-44 stabilizes HLA-E expression and inhibits cytolysis mediated by natural killer cells. The American Journal of Pathology. 2005;166(2):443-453

[58] Castelli EC et al. Insights into HLA-G genetics provided by worldwide haplotype diversity. Frontiers in Immunology. 2014;5:476

[59] Hviid TV et al. Co-dominant expression of the HLA-G gene and various forms of alternatively spliced HLA-G mRNA in human first trimester trophoblast. Human Immunology. 1998;59(2):87-98

[60] Ishitani A, Geraghty DE. Alternative splicing of HLA-G transcripts yields proteins with primary structures resembling both class I and class II antigens. Proceedings of the National Academy of Sciences of the United States of America. 1992;89(9): 3947-3951

[61] Rizzo R et al. Matrix metalloproteinase-2 (MMP-2) generates soluble HLA-G1 by cell surface proteolytic shedding. Molecular and Cellular Biochemistry. 2013;381(1-2):243-255

[62] HoWangYin K-Y et al. Multimeric structures of HLA-G isoforms function through differential binding to LILRB receptors. Cellular and Molecular Life Sciences. 2012;69(23):4041-4049

[63] Dong Y et al. Soluble nonclassical HLA generated by the metalloproteinase pathway. Human Immunology. 2003;64(8):802-810

[64] Gonen-Gross T et al. The CD85J/ leukocyte inhibitory receptor-1 distinguishes between conformed and beta 2-microglobulin-free HLA-G molecules. Journal of Immunology. 2005;175(8):4866-4874

[65] Paul P et al. Identification of HLA-G7 as a new splice variant of the HLA-G mRNA and expression of soluble HLA-G5, -G6, and -G7 transcripts in human transfected cells. Human Immunology. 2000;**61**(11):1138-1149

[66] Riteau B et al. HLA-G2, -G3, and -G4 isoforms expressed as nonmature cell surface glycoproteins inhibit NK and antigen-specific CTL cytolysis. Journal of Immunology. 2001;**166**(8):5018-5026

[67] Lila N et al. Implication of HLA-G molecule in heart-graft acceptance. Lancet. 2000;**355**(9221):2138

[68] Shiroishi M et al. Structural basis for recognition of the nonclassical MHC molecule HLA-G by the leukocyte Ig-like receptor B2 (LILRB2/LIR2/ILT4/CD85d). Proceedings of the National Academy of Sciences of the United States of America. 2006;**103**(44):16412-16417

[69] Diehl M et al. Nonclassical HLA-G molecules are classical peptide presenters. Current Biology. 1996;**6**(3):305-314

[70] Celik AA et al. HLA-G peptide preferences change in transformed cells: Impact on the binding motif. Immunogenetics. 2018;**70**(8): 485-494

[71] Ellis SA, Palmer MS, McMichael AJ. Human trophoblast and the choriocarcinoma cell line BeWo express a truncated HLA Class I molecule. Journal of Immunology. 1990;**144**(2):731-735

[72] Mallet V et al. HLA-G in the human thymus: A subpopulation of medullary epithelial but not CD83(+) dendritic cells expresses HLA-G as a membrane-bound and soluble protein. International Immunology. 1999;**11**(6):889-898

[73] Ito T et al. Immunology of the human nail apparatus: The nail matrix is a site of relative immune privilege. The Journal of Investigative Dermatology. 2005;**125**(6):1139-1148

[74] Cirulli V et al. The class I HLA repertoire of pancreatic islets comprises the nonclassical class Ib antigen HLA-G. Diabetes. 2006;**55**(5):1214-1222

[75] Menier C et al. Erythroblasts secrete the nonclassical HLA-G molecule from primitive to definitive hematopoiesis. Blood. 2004;**104**(10):3153-3160

[76] Carosella ED et al. Beyond the increasing complexity of the immunomodulatory HLA-G molecule. Blood. 2008;**111**(10):4862-4870

[77] Carosella ED et al. HLA-G: From biology to clinical benefits. Trends in Immunology. 2008;**29**(3):125-132

[78] Rizzo R et al. HLA-G molecules in autoimmune diseases and infections. Frontiers in Immunology. 2014;**5**:592

[79] Juch H et al. HLA class I expression in the human placenta. Wiener Medizinische Wochenschrift. 2012;**162**(9-10):196-200

[80] Fournel S et al. Cutting edge: soluble HLA-G1 triggers CD95/CD95 ligand-mediated apoptosis in activated CD8+ cells by interacting with CD8. Journal of Immunology. 2000;**164**(12):6100-6104

[81] Kovats S et al. A class I antigen, HLA-G, expressed in human trophoblasts. Science. 1990;**248**(4952):220-223

[82] Apps R et al. Human leucocyte antigen (HLA) expression of primary trophoblast cells and placental cell lines, determined using single antigen beads to characterize allotype specificities of anti-HLA antibodies. Immunology. 2009;**127**(1):26-39

[83] Bainbridge DR, Ellis SA, Sargent IL. HLA-G suppresses proliferation of CD4(+) T-lymphocytes. Journal of Reproductive Immunology. 2000;**48**(1):17-26

[84] Li C et al. HLA-G homodimer-induced cytokine secretion through HLA-G receptors on human decidual macrophages and natural killer cells. Proceedings of the National Academy of Sciences of the United States of America. 2009;**106**(14):5767-5772

[85] Naji A et al. Binding of HLA-G to ITIM-bearing Ig-like transcript 2 receptor suppresses B cell responses. Journal of Immunology. 2014;**192**(4):1536-1546

[86] Rouas-Freiss N et al. The alpha1 domain of HLA-G1 and HLA-G2 inhibits cytotoxicity induced by natural killer cells: Is HLA-G the public ligand for natural killer cell inhibitory receptors? Proceedings of the National Academy of Sciences of the United States of America. 1997;**94**(10):5249-5254

[87] Rajagopalan S, Long EO. A human histocompatibility leukocyte antigen (HLA)-G–specific receptor expressed on all natural killer cells. The Journal of Experimental Medicine. 1999;**189**(7):1093-1100

[88] Hunt JS et al. A commentary on gestational programming and functions of HLA-G in pregnancy. Placenta. 2007;**28**:S57-S63

[89] Clements CS et al. Crystal structure of HLA-G: A nonclassical MHC class I molecule expressed at the fetal-maternal interface. Proceedings of the National Academy of Sciences of the United States of America. 2005;**102**(9):3360-3365

[90] Jabrane-Ferrat N, Siewiera J. The up side of decidual natural killer cells: New developments in immunology

of pregnancy. Immunology. 2014;**141**(4):490-497

[91] Tilburgs T et al. The HLA-G cycle provides for both NK tolerance and immunity at the maternal–fetal interface. Proceedings of the National Academy of Sciences of the United States of America. 2015;**112**(43):13312-13317

[92] Ferreira LMR et al. HLA-G: At the Interface of maternal-Fetal tolerance. Trends in Immunology. 2017;**38**(4):272-286

[93] Riteau B et al. HLA-G inhibits the allogeneic proliferative response. Journal of Reproductive Immunology. 1999;**43**(2):203-211

[94] LeMaoult J et al. HLA-G1-expressing antigen-presenting cells induce immunosuppressive CD4+ T cells. Proceedings of the National Academy of Sciences of the United States of America. 2004;**101**(18):7064-7069

[95] Liang S et al. Modulation of dendritic cell differentiation by HLA-G and ILT4 requires the IL-6-STAT3 signaling pathway. Proceedings of the National Academy of Sciences of the United States of America. 2008;**105**(24):8357-8362

[96] Gregori S et al. Differentiation of type 1 T regulatory cells (Tr1) by tolerogenic DC-10 requires the IL-10-dependent ILT4/HLA-G pathway. Blood. 2010;**116**(6):935-944

[97] Selmani Z et al. Human leukocyte antigen-G5 secretion by human mesenchymal stem cells is required to suppress T lymphocyte and natural killer function and to induce CD4+ CD25^{high}FOXP3+ regulatory T cells. Stem Cells. 2008;**26**(1):212-222

[98] Carosella ED, Gregori S, Lemaoult J. The tolerogenic

interplay(s) among HLA-G, myeloid APCs, and regulatory cells. Blood. 2011;**118**(25):6499-6505

[99] Shiroishi M et al. Human inhibitory receptors Ig-like transcript 2 (ILT2) and ILT4 compete with CD8 for MHC class I binding and bind preferentially to HLA-G. Proceedings of the National Academy of Sciences of the United States of America. 2003;**100**(15):8856-8861

[100] Nam G et al. Crystal structures of the two membrane-proximal Ig-like domains (D3D4) of LILRB1/B2: Alternative models for their involvement in peptide-HLA binding. Protein & Cell. 2013;**4**(10):761-770

[101] Morandi F et al. Recent advances in our understanding of HLA-G biology: Lessons from a wide spectrum of human diseases. Journal of Immunology Research. 2016;**2016**

[102] Zheng J et al. Human leukocyte antigen G is associated with esophageal squamous cell carcinoma progression and poor prognosis. Immunology Letters. 2014;**161**(1):13-19

[103] Guo Z-Y et al. Predictive value of HLA-G and HLA-E in the prognosis of colorectal cancer patients. Cellular Immunology. 2015;**293**(1):10-16

[104] Sebti Y et al. Expression of functional soluble human leucocyte antigen-G molecules in lymphoproliferative disorders. British Journal of Haematology. 2007;**138**(2):202-212

[105] Leleu X et al. Total soluble HLA class I and soluble HLA-G in multiple myeloma and monoclonal gammopathy of undetermined significance. Clinical Cancer Research: An Official Journal of the American Association for Cancer Research. 2005;**11**(20):7297-7303

[106] Yan W-H et al. Significance of tumour cell HLA-G5/-G6 isoform expression in discrimination for adenocarcinoma from squamous cell carcinoma in lung cancer patients. Journal of Cellular and Molecular Medicine. 2015;**19**(4):778-785

[107] Lazarte J et al. 10-Year Experience with HLA-G in Heart Transplantation. Human Immunology. 2018;**79**(8):587-593

[108] Sheshgiri R et al. Myocardial HLA-G reliably indicates a low risk of acute cellular rejection in heart transplant recipients. The Journal of Heart and Lung Transplantation: The Official Publication of the International Society for Heart Transplantation. 2008;**27**(5):522-527

[109] Brugière O et al. Immunohistochemical study of HLA-G expression in lung transplant recipients. American Journal of Transplantation: Official Journal of the American Society of Transplantation and the American Society of Transplant Surgeons. 2009;**9**(6):1427-1438

[110] Créput C et al. Human leukocyte antigen-G (HLA-G) expression in biliary epithelial cells is associated with allograft acceptance in liver-kidney transplantation. Journal of Hepatology. 2003;**39**(4):587-594

[111] Sheshgiri R et al. Association between HLA-G expression and C4d staining in cardiac transplantation. Transplantation. 2010;**89**(4):480-481

[112] Misra MK et al. Association of HLA-G promoter and 14-bp insertion-deletion variants with acute allograft rejection and end-stage renal disease. Tissue Antigens. 2013;**82**(5):317-326

[113] Lemaoult J et al. Synthetic HLA-G proteins for therapeutic use in transplantation. FASEB Journal: Official Publication of the Federation

of American Societies for Experimental Biology. 2013;**27**(9):3643-3651

[114] Torres MI et al. New advances in coeliac disease: Serum and intestinal expression of HLA-G. International Immunology. 2006;**18**(5):713-718

[115] Aractingi S et al. HLA-G and NK receptor are expressed in psoriatic skin: A possible pathway for regulating infiltrating T cells? The American Journal of Pathology. 2001;**159**(1):71-77

[116] Gazit E et al. HLA-G is associated with pemphigus vulgaris in Jewish patients. Human Immunology. 2004;**65**(1):39-46

[117] Rizzo R et al. HLA-G may predict the disease course in patients with early rheumatoid arthritis. Human Immunology. 2013;**74**(4):425-432

[118] Rizzo R et al. Different production of soluble HLA-G antigens by peripheral blood mononuclear cells in ulcerative colitis and Crohn's disease: A noninvasive diagnostic tool? Inflammatory Bowel Diseases. 2008;**14**(1):100-105

[119] Zelante A et al. Therapy modifies HLA-G secretion differently in Crohn's disease and ulcerative colitis patients. Inflammatory Bowel Diseases. 2011;**17**(8):E94-E95

[120] Yari F et al. Expression of HLA-G in the skin of patients with pemphigus vulgaris. Iranian Journal of Allergy, Asthma, and Immunology. 2008;**7**(1):7-12

[121] Wiendl H et al. Expression of the immune-tolerogenic major histocompatibility molecule HLA-G in multiple sclerosis: Implications for CNS immunity. Brain: A Journal of Neurology. 2005;**128**(Pt 11):2689-2704

[122] Huang Y-H et al. Specific central nervous system recruitment

of HLA-G(+) regulatory T cells in multiple sclerosis. Annals of Neurology. 2009;**66**(2):171-183

[123] Huang Y-H et al. T cell suppression by naturally occurring HLA-G-expressing regulatory CD4+ T cells is IL-10-dependent and reversible. Journal of Leukocyte Biology. 2009;**86**(2):273-281

[124] Feger U et al. HLA-G expression defines a novel regulatory T-cell subset present in human peripheral blood and sites of inflammation. Blood. 2007;**110**(2):568-577

[125] Waschbisch A et al. Evaluation of soluble HLA-G as a biomarker for multiple sclerosis. Neurology. 2011;**77**(6):596-598

[126] Amiot L, Vu N, Samson M. Immunomodulatory properties of HLA-G in infectious diseases. Journal of Immunology Research. 2014;**2014**:298569

[127] Reddy RC et al. Sepsis-induced immunosuppression: From bad to worse. Immunologic Research. 2001;**24**(3):273-287

[128] Robbins JR et al. Tissue barriers of the human placenta to infection with toxoplasma gondii. Infection and Immunity. 2012;**80**(1):418-428

[129] Sadissou I et al. High plasma levels of HLA-G are associated with low birth weight and with an increased risk of malaria in infancy. Malaria Journal. 2014;**13**:312

[130] Wilson EB, Brooks DG. The role of IL-10 in regulating immunity to persistent viral infections. Current Topics in Microbiology and Immunology. 2011;**350**:39-65

[131] Onno M et al. Modulation of HLA-G antigens expression by human cytomegalovirus: Specific

induction in activated macrophages harboring human cytomegalovirus infection. Journal of Immunology. 2000;**164**(12):6426-6434

[132] Shi W-W et al. Plasma soluble human leukocyte antigen-G expression is a potential clinical biomarker in patients with hepatitis B virus infection. Human Immunology. 2011;**72**(11):1068-1073

[133] Weng P-J et al. Elevation of plasma soluble human leukocyte antigen-G in patients with chronic hepatitis C virus infection. Human Immunology. 2011;**72**(5):406-411

[134] Souto FJD et al. Liver HLA-G expression is associated with multiple clinical and histopathological forms of chronic hepatitis B virus infection. Journal of Viral Hepatitis. 2011;**18**(2):102-105

[135] Amiot L et al. Expression of HLA-G by mast cells is associated with hepatitis C virus-induced liver fibrosis. Journal of Hepatology. 2014;**60**(2):245-252

[136] Lozano JM et al. Monocytes and T lymphocytes in HIV-1-positive patients express HLA-G molecule. AIDS. 2002;**16**(3):347-351

[137] Cabello A et al. HAART induces the expression of HLA-G on peripheral monocytes in HIV-1 infected individuals. Human Immunology. 2003;**64**(11):1045-1049

[138] Lajoie J et al. Genetic variants in nonclassical major histocompatibility complex class I human leukocyte antigen (HLA)-E and HLA-G molecules are associated with susceptibility to heterosexual acquisition of HIV-1. The Journal of Infectious Diseases. 2006;**193**(2):298-301

[139] Matte C et al. Functionally active HLA-G polymorphisms are associated with the risk of heterosexual HIV-1

infection in African women. AIDS. 2004;**18**(3):427-431

[140] Elsner HA, Blasczyk R. Immunogenetics of HLA null alleles: implications for blood stem cell transplantation. Tissue Antigens. 2004;**64**(6):687-95

[141] Geraghty DE. Human leukocyte antigen F (HLA-F). An expressed HLA gene composed of a class I coding sequence linked to a novel transcribed repetitive element. Journal of Experimental Medicine. 1990;**171**(1):1-18

[142] Geraghty DE, Koller BH, Orr HT. A human major histocompatibility complex class I gene that encodes a protein with a shortened cytoplasmic segment. Proceedings of the National Academy of Sciences of the United States of America. 1987;**84**(24):9145-9149

[143] Boyle LH et al. Selective export of HLA-F by its cytoplasmic tail. Journal of Immunology. 2006;**176**(11):6464-6472

[144] Dulberger CL et al. Human leukocyte antigen F presents peptides and regulates immunity through interactions with NK cell receptors. Immunity. 2017;**46**(6):1018-1029 e7

[145] Lee N, Ishitani A, Geraghty DE. HLA-F is a surface marker on activated lymphocytes. European Journal of Immunology. 2010;**40**(8):2308-2318

[146] Ishitani A et al. Protein expression and peptide binding suggest unique and interacting functional roles for HLA-E, F, and G in maternal-placental immune recognition. The Journal of Immunology. 2003;**171**(3):1376-1384

[147] Burrows CK et al. Expression quantitative trait locus mapping studies in mid-secretory phase endometrial cells identifies HLA-F and TAP2 as

Fecundability-associated genes. PLoS
Genetics. 2016;**12**(7):e1005858

[148] Goodridge JP et al. HLA-F
and MHC class I open conformers
are ligands for NK cell Ig-like
receptors. Journal of Immunology.
2013;**191**(7):3553-3562

[149] Lin A et al. HLA-F expression is a
prognostic factor in patients with non-
small-cell lung cancer. Lung Cancer.
2011;**74**(3):504-509

[150] Zhang X et al. Alteration of HLA-F
and HLA I antigen expression in the
tumor is associated with survival in
patients with esophageal squamous cell
carcinoma. International Journal of
Cancer. 2013;**132**(1):82-89

[151] Ishigami S et al. Clinical-
pathological implication of human
leukocyte antigen-F-positive gastric
adenocarcinoma. The Journal of
Surgical Research. 2013;**184**(2):802-806

[152] Harada A et al. Clinical implication
of human leukocyte antigen (HLA)-F
expression in breast cancer. Pathology
International. 2015;**65**(11):569-574

Chapter 3

Psychoneuroimmunology and Genetics

Rama P. Vempati and Hemakumar M. Reddy

Abstract

Psychoneuroimmunology is a study that investigates the interaction between human emotions and the immune system, which is mediated by the endocrine and nervous systems. The nervous and immune systems maintain extensive communication, including communication to lymphoid organs from deep-rooted sympathetic and parasympathetic nerves. Genetic factors are responsible for individual variation in emotional reactivity, and neuroendocrine stress responses were shown by earlier studies in humans. Several gene-environment studies have shown that long-term effects of stress are being moderated by genetic variations in the hypothalamic-pituitary-adrenal (HPA) axis. There is a large interindividual variability of HPA axis stress reactivity on variants of the glucocorticoid (GR) or mineralocorticoid receptor genes, and it documents a sex-specific association between different GR gene polymorphisms and salivary cortisol responses to acute psychosocial stress. In conclusion, many kinds of mind-body behavioral interventions are effective in improving mood, quality of life, reducing stress, and anxiety, thereby altering neuroendocrine and immune functions, and ultimately altering the genetic aberrations. However, the question remains as to whether these latter effects are sufficiently large or last long enough to contribute to health benefits, or if they are even relevant to the development of a disease.

Keywords: psychoneuroimmunology, immunology and genetics, emotional stress, genetic factors involved in stress, epigenetics involved in stress

1. Psychoneuroimmunology

Psychoneuroimmunology is an area that examines the interaction between human emotions and the immune system, which is mediated by the endocrine and nervous system. The brain controls the immune system by hardwiring sympathetic and parasympathetic nerves to lymphoid organs. Further neuroendocrine hormones such as a corticotropin-releasing hormone or substance P regulate cytokine balance. The immune system controls some brain activities such as sleep and body temperature. Based on anatomical and a close functional connection, the nervous and immune systems act in a very mutual way. Over recent decades, reasonable evidence has emerged that these brain-to-immune interactions are highly modulated by psychological factors which influence immunity and immune system-mediated disease [1].

The nervous and immune systems maintain extensive communication, including communication to lymphoid organs from deep-rooted sympathetic and parasympathetic nerves. Acetylcholine, norepinephrine, vasoactive intestinal peptide, substance P, and histamine such as neurotransmitters modulate immune activity. Corticotropin-releasing factor, leptin, and alpha-melanocyte-stimulating hormone such neuroendocrine hormones regulate cytokine balance. The brain activity mainly body temperature, sleep, and feeding behavior is influenced by the immune system. The major histocompatibility complex directs T cells to immunogenic molecules held in its cleft and also controls the development of neuronal connections. Neurobiologists and immunologists are exploring common ideas like the synapse to understand properties such as memory which is shared between these two systems [2].

Both neuronal (direct sympathetic innervation of the lymphoid organ) and neuroendocrine (hypothalamic-pituitary-adrenal axis) pathways are involved in the control of the humoral and cellular immune responses. There is a recent evidence on the immunosuppressive effect of acetylcholine-secreting neurons of the parasympathetic nervous system which influences the central nervous system primarily through cytokines. Neuroimmune signal molecules such as hormones, neurotransmitters, neuropeptides, cytokines, or their receptors enable mutual neuroimmune communication. Subcellular and molecular mechanisms of cytokine-neuropeptide/neurotransmitter interactions were extensively investigated. At the neuroanatomical level, neuroimmune communication in the role of discrete brain areas related to emotionality has been established. Immuno-enhancement, including the antitumor cytotoxic activity and antiviral activity, related to the "brain reward system," limbic structures, and neocortex, offers a new direction for therapy in immune disorders [3].

2. Immunology and genetics

Genetic predisposition is important for this immune function. Stress-mediated inflammation is a common feature of many hereditary disorders, due to the proteotoxic effects of mutant proteins. Harmful mutant proteins can induce dysregulated IL-1β production and inflammation. Depressive disorders are often accompanied by profound changes in immunity. Clinical observations in depression disorders showed that immune dysfunction is the main cause of increased risks in other oncological, inflammatory, and infectious diseases. Immunological reactions in psychoemotional stress play an important role. Studying Antidepressant-Sensitive Catalepsy (ASC) in mice showed a decrease in IgM immune responses and sensitivity to the administration of antidepressants. Unlike their non-depressive parental CBA strains, ASC lines show the difference in T-lymphocyte distribution and changes in IgG and IgM immune responses, low antibody production, abnormal CD4+ T-cell content in blood and spleen, and variations in CD4+/CD8+ T-cell ratio [4].

Stress-induced inflammation is a key pathogenic factor in inherited diseases and autoinflammatory syndromes. The stress contributes severity of the symptoms in these diseases. A study showed the correlation among basal stress, disease severity, and antioxidant response in two different cryopyrin-associated periodic syndrome (CAPS) patients sharing same nucleotide-binding domain, leucine-rich-containing family, pyrin domain-containing 3 (NLRP3) mutation [5]. Hence, similar stress-related mechanisms may operate in other genetic diseases, where inflammation causes disease progression and mutant protein present in monocytes. Improving the responses to stress represents a promising therapeutic opportunity for this kind of serious diseases, while considering the genetic factor (individual tolerance levels) may play a major role.

3. Molecular mechanisms of emotional stress

Identification of mechanisms underlying a dysregulation of major components of the stress response system is a very challenging task as it involves complex cellular interactions at the level of different organs and systems. One of the main features of the stress response is the activation of the hypothalamic-pituitary-adrenal axis (HPA) [6]. The main regions of the brain that shows stress response are hippocampus, amygdala, and prefrontal cortex. Decreased activity and neuronal atrophy in the hippocampus and in the prefrontal cortex, as well as increased activity and neuronal growth in the amygdala, are involved in post-traumatic stress disorder (PTSD) [6]. The changes that stress induces mainly affect the levels of cortisol and catecholamines (epinephrine, norepinephrine, dopamine). Catecholamines are released shortly after stress onset and go back to normal levels upon stress termination. Glucocorticoids act by binding to two types of receptors—mineralocorticoid receptors (MR) and glucocorticoid receptors (GR). Molecular mechanisms involving this stress response are genetic, epigenetic, and immunological nature.

4. Hormonal and immunological factors in stress response

The primary hormonal end product of the HPA axis is cortisol. A longitudinal study of 358 Dutch adolescents with a mean age of 15 years over 3 years showed that cortisol awakening response (CAR) moderated the effects of depressive symptoms on violent adult outcomes. The results showed that depressive symptoms were positively associated with violent outcomes when CAR levels are low [7].

Mental and physical stress can suppress the immune system in both humans and animals. Chronic stress-induced alterations in immune responses could result from increased cell death and apoptosis or decreased cell proliferation. It is well known that exhausting physical activity and mental stress lead to immunosuppression of the immune system by steroid hormone regulation. Chronic stress significantly enhances corticosterone production and induces lymphocyte apoptosis [8, 9]. Stress hormones like cortisol play a fundamental role in regulating immune responses and the balance of T helper (Th) 1 and Th2 cytokines, thereby modulating the susceptibility of various immune-related disorders. Toll-like receptors (TLRs) play a key role in modulating immune responses, cell apoptosis, and cell survival. Among 11 known TLRs in mammals, TLR9 plays a major role in chronic stress-induced immune suppression by modulating corticosteroid levels [10].

Psychosocial stressors increase peripheral cytokine production, a potentially important factor in the development of depression or anxiety [11, 12]. Subsets of patients with the major depressive disorder (MDD) and post-traumatic stress disorder have higher levels of multiple inflammatory markers, including the cytokine interleukin 6 (IL-6) [11, 13]. Preexisting differences in the sensitivity of an individual's peripheral immune system like cytokine interleukin 6 (IL-6) dictates their subsequent vulnerability or resilience to social stress [14].

5. Genetic factors involved in stress

Molecular studies of the stress phenomenon have found some genes which are differentially expressed in stressed individuals and control subjects. Studies involving effect at individual genes as well as genome-wide studies at cellular, tissue, and individual levels are reported.

A study of DNA microarray from circulating leucocytes showed that the stress causes some genes upregulated and some other genes downregulated. The downregulated genes are mainly related to apoptosis, cell cycle inhibitors, NF-KB inhibitor (Apo J), and antiproliferative cytokines. The upregulated genes are involved in cell cycle activation, and enzymes involved in nucleic acid biosynthesis and proteins. Other upregulated genes are transcription factors that control chromatin structure and cell growth [15]. The transcription factor that controls many of these genes is NF-KB. Hence, NF-KB plays a key role in the cellular stress response.

Researchers have attempted to attribute genetic variation among individuals to their neuroendocrine responsiveness to environmental stimuli like stress by studying how the immune system interacts with the nervous and endocrine systems and, together, how they impact upon the course and outcome of disease [16]. As early as 1992, Gatz et al. studied the importance of genes and environments on the symptoms of depression [17].

Genetic factors are responsible for individual variation in emotional reactivity, and neuroendocrine stress responses were shown by family and twin studies in humans and by the study of inbred strains and selection experiments in animals [18]. A twin study revealed the significant genetic impact on the cortisol awakening response with heritability estimates between 0.40 and 0.48 for the mean cortisol increase after awakening and the area under the curve, respectively [19]. An increased cortisol awakening response in individuals reporting chronic stress includes social stress and lack of social recognition [19].

Several gene-environment studies have shown that long-term effects of stress are being moderated by genetic variations in the hypothalamic-pituitary-adrenal (HPA) axis. Studies by Wust et al. investigated contribution of large interindividual variability of HPA axis stress reactivity on variants of the glucocorticoid or mineralocorticoid receptor genes and documented a sex-specific association between different GR gene polymorphisms and salivary cortisol responses to acute psychosocial stress [20]. Single-nucleotide polymorphisms (SNPs) associated with stress vulnerability and resilience are found in the GR (e.g., through regulation by the FK506 binding protein 5 [FKBP5]), the corticotropin-releasing hormone factor receptor 1 (CRHR1), and the MR genes [21].

The genetic component is often complex in these studies and involves several genes and, hence, should study the quantitative trait loci (QTL). It is easy to study QTL in plants and animals where you can easily get the inbred lines where the genetic makeup is similar among individuals. Quantitative genetic analysis to behavioral responses to environmental challenges like stress in humans is done mainly on the large cohorts of families and twins.

Another approach is the utilization of genome-wide association studies (GWAS) that would facilitate identification of new genes involved in stress development and elucidate the molecular pathways which are dysregulated. In contrast to candidate gene studies that are based on prior biological knowledge, in GWASs common variants across the whole genome are screened concerning the contributing genes. GWASs for human stress-related phenotypes are rare [21]. A meta-analysis on plasma cortisol levels in 12,597 participants found a genome-wide association of SNPs in the SERPINA6/SERPINA1 locus. GWAS and individual gene studies are often underpowered owing to smaller sample sizes. There is a need to test whether the identified candidate genes appear to be nominally significant in the GWASs in larger samples [21].

6. Epigenetics involved in stress

Even though genome is the blueprint for biological activity, the epigenome adds another layer on top of the genome and serves to modulate gene expression in response to environmental cues. Epigenetic modification induced by environmental factors could influence the development of chronic pain by modulating genomic expression of one or more biological systems associated with pain and psychological stressors. Recent studies demonstrate that adverse psychosocial environments like stress can affect gene expression by altering the epigenetic pattern of DNA methylation, chromatin structure by histone modifications, and noncoding RNA expression [22].

Most of the epigenetic studies employ animal models at early life experiences that demonstrate epigenetic modification that occurs in response to stressors, which alter the developing epigenome in the hippocampus. Some studies evaluate epigenetic modification using adult models of stress and depression as well as consideration of the role of epigenetics in resilient versus susceptible phenotypes. Adverse events such as stress or maltreatment at early stages of development can more readily trigger epigenetic alterations which can adversely affect physiological function and behavior in adult life. Studies involving human samples from different models like suicide victims with and without child abuse, prenatal depression, and post-traumatic stress disorder showed altered DNA methylation patterns at the glucocorticoid receptor gene (NR3C1) [22]. The salivary cortisol response which in turn leads to altered central regulation of the HPA axis consequent to maternal depressed mood. Epigenetic changes due to stress affected the gene expression of several genes including estrogen receptor alpha (ER-A), trichostatin (TSA), N-methyl-D-aspartate (NMDA), nerve growth factor-inducible protein-A (NGFI-A), arginine vasopressin (AVP), brain-derived neurotrophic factor (BDNF), and cyclic-AMP response element-binding protein (CREB) [22]. Telomere shortening is one of the molecular indicators as an epigenetic effect on stress and chronic pain [23].

7. Biomarkers for diagnosis and treatment of stress

The hypothalamus-pituitary-adrenal axis (HPA axis) is a vital part of the human stress response system. The endocrine marker cortisol is a useful index of HPA axis activity, and it shows good intraindividual stability across time and appears to uncover subtle changes in HPA regulation. Cortisol activity and the response are important biological indicators of emotional and behavioral responses to environmental stressors. Low cortisol activity is hypothesized to be linked to antisocial behaviors [24]. Several studies demonstrated the role of age and gender; endogenous and exogenous sex steroid levels; pregnancy, lactation, and breastfeeding; smoking, coffee, and alcohol consumption; as well as dietary energy supply in salivary cortisol responses to acute stress [25]. Salivary cortisol levels are a reliable measure of HPA axis adaptation to stress and hence are a useful and valid biomarker in stress research [26].

The knowledge of the molecular bases of genetic variability points to the biochemical pathways responsible for the differences in stress responses will allow the development of new therapeutic strategies for pathological conditions [18]. Interventions aimed at manipulating the epigenome are a real and promising possibility to circumvent the stress-related psychoneuroimmunology disorders. Epigenetic and telomere changes may offer an array of targets that can be exploited for prevention and treatment interventions [27].

In conclusion, many kinds of mind-body behavioral interventions are effective in improving mood, quality of life, reducing stress, and anxiety, thereby altering neuroendocrine and immune functions, and ultimately altering the genetic aberrations. However, the question remains as to whether these latter effects are sufficiently large or last long enough to contribute to health benefits or if they are even relevant to the development of a disease. Unfortunately, there is no strong body of evidence that supports the clinical correlation between psychoneuroimmunology and genetics and reaping the health benefits through behavioral interventions.

Author details

Rama P. Vempati[1*] and Hemakumar M. Reddy[2]

1 Clinical Safety Sciences, Sunnyvale, CA, USA

2 Department of Molecular Biology, Cell Biology and Biochemistry, Brown University Division of Biology and Medicine, Providence, RI, USA

*Address all correspondence to: rpvempati@gmail.com

IntechOpen

© 2019 The Author(s). Licensee IntechOpen. This chapter is distributed under the terms of the Creative Commons Attribution License (http://creativecommons.org/licenses/by/3.0), which permits unrestricted use, distribution, and reproduction in any medium, provided the original work is properly cited. (cc) BY

References

[1] Ziemssen T, Kern S. Psychoneuroimmunology—Cross-talk between the immune and nervous systems. Journal of Neurology. 2007;**254**(Suppl 2):8-11

[2] Steinman L. Elaborate interactions between the immune and nervous systems. Nature Immunology. 2004;**5**(6):575-581

[3] Wrona D. Neural-immune interactions: An integrative view of the bidirectional relationship between the brain and immune systems. Journal of Neuroimmunology. 2006;**172**(1-2):38-58

[4] Idova GV, Al'perina EL, Gevorgyan MM, et al. T-lymphocyte subpopulation composition and the immune response in depression-like behavior in ASC mice. Neuroscience and Behavioral Physiology. 2013;**43**:946

[5] Carta S, Semino C, Sitia R, et al. Dysregulated IL-1β secretion in autoinflammatory diseases: A matter of stress? Frontiers in Immunology. 2017;**8**:345

[6] Feodorova YN, Sarafian VS. Psychological stress—Cellular and molecular mechanisms. Folia Medica. 2012;**54**(3):5-13

[7] Yu R, Branje S, Meeus W, et al. Depression, violence, and cortisol awakening response: A 3-year longitudinal study in adolescents. Psychological Medicine. 2018 Jul 17:1-8. doi: 10.1017/S0033291718001654. [Epub ahead of print]

[8] Ader R, Cohen N. Psychoneuroimmunology: Conditioning and stress. Annual Review of Psychology. 1993;**44**:53-85

[9] Wang KX, Shi Y, Denhardt DT. Osteopontin regulates hindlimb-unloading-induced lymphoid organ atrophy and weight loss by modulating corticosteroid production. Proceedings of the National Academy of Sciences of the United States of America. 2007;**104**(37):14777-14782

[10] Li H, Zhao J, Chen M, et al. Toll-like receptor 9 is required for chronic stress-induced immune suppression. Neuroimmunomodulation. 2014;**21**:1-7

[11] Maes M et al. Leukocytosis, monocytosis and neutrophilia: Hallmarks of severe depression. Journal of Psychiatric Research. 1992;**26**(2):125-134

[12] Fagundes CP, Glaser R, Hwang BS, et al. Depressive symptoms enhance stress-induced inflammatory responses. Brain, Behavior, and Immunity. 2013;**31**:172-176

[13] Cole SW et al. Computational identification of gene-social environment interaction at the human IL6 locus. Proceedings of the National Academy of Sciences of the United States of America. 2010;**107**(12):5681-5686

[14] Hodes GE, Pfau ML, Leboeuf M, et al. Individual differences in the peripheral immune system promote resilience versus susceptibility to social stress. Proceedings of the National Academy of Sciences of the United States of America. 2014;**111**(45):16136-16141

[15] Cole SW, Hawkley LC, Arevalo JM, et al. Social regulation of gene expression in human leukocytes. Genome Biology. 2007;**8**(9):R189

[16] Bonneau RH, Morme'de P, George P, et al. A genetic basis for neuroendocrine–immune interactions.

Brain, Behavior, and Immunity. 1998;**12**:83-89

[17] Gatz M, Pedersen NL, Plomin R, et al. Importance of shared genes and shared environments for symptoms of depression in older adults. Journal of Abnormal Psychology. 1992;**101**:701-708

[18] Mormède P, Courvoisier H, Ramos A, et al. Molecular genetic approaches to investigate individual variations in behavioral and neuroendocrine stress responses. Psychoneuroendocrinology. 2002;**27**(5):563-583

[19] Wüst S, Federenko I, Hellhammer DH, et al. Genetic factors, perceived chronic stress, and the free cortisol response to awakening. Psychoneuroendocrinology. 2000;**25**(7):707-720

[20] Wust S, Van Rossum EF, Federenko IS, et al. Common polymorphisms in glucocorticoid receptor gene are associated with adrenocortical responses to psychosocial stress. The Journal of Clinical Endocrinology and Metabolism. 2004;**89**:565-573

[21] Nees F, Witt SH, Flor H. Neurogenetic approaches to stress and fear in humans as pathophysiological mechanisms for posttraumatic stress disorder. Biological Psychiatry. 2018;**83**(10):810-820

[22] Mathews HL, Janusek LW. Epigenetics and psychoneuroimmunology: Mechanisms and models. Brain, behavior, and immunity. 2011;**25**(1):25-39

[23] Epel E, Lin J, Dhabhar FS, Wolkowitz OM, et al. Dynamics of telomerase activity in response to acute psychological stress. Brain, Behavior, and Immunity. 2010;**24**:531-539

[24] Raine A. Biosocial studies of antisocial and violent behavior in children and adults: A review. Journal of Abnormal Child Psychology. 2002;**30**:311-326

[25] Kudielka BM, Hellhammer DH, Wüst S. Why do we respond so differently? Reviewing determinants of human salivary cortisol responses to challenge. Psychoneuroendocrinology. 2009;**34**(1):2-18

[26] Hellhammer DH, Wüst S, Kudielka BM. Salivary cortisol as a biomarker in stress research. Psychoneuroendocrinology. 2009;**34**(2):163-171

[27] Sibille KT, Witek-Janusek L, Mathews HL, et al. Telomeres and epigenetics: Potential relevance to chronic pain. Pain. 2012;**153**(9):1789-1793

Chapter 4

Immunoassay Techniques Highlighting Biomarkers in Immunogenetic Diseases

Emilia Manole, Alexandra E. Bastian, Ionela D. Popescu,
Carolina Constantin, Simona Mihai, Gisela F. Gaina,
Elena Codrici and Monica T. Neagu

Abstract

Diagnosis of autoimmune diseases is crucial for the clinician and the patient alike. The immunoassay techniques most commonly used for this purpose are immunohistochemistry, ELISA, and Western blotting. For the detection of more specific biomarkers or the discovery of new ones for diagnostic purposes and as therapeutic targets, microarray techniques are increasingly used, for example, protein microarray, Luminex, and in recent years, surface plasmon resonance imaging. All of these technologies have undergone changes over time, making them easier to use. Similar technologies have been invented but responding to specific requirements for both diagnostic and research purposes. The goals are to study more analytes in the same sample, in a shorter time, and with increased accuracy. The reproducibility and reliability of the results are also a target pursued by manufacturers. In this chapter, we present these technologies and their utility in the diagnosis of immunogenetic diseases.

Keywords: immunoassay, protein biomarkers, autoimmune diseases, IHC, ELISA, WB, protein microarray, SPRi, Luminex

1. Introduction

An autoimmune pathology occurs when the immune system loses its ability to distinguish between its own cells and nonself cells, inducing the attack of self-tissue. This mechanism involves both the environmental factors and the genetic predisposition of the individual.

Proteomic technologies identify and separate different proteins of interest from biological samples, thus enabling their characterization as biomarkers, establishing their interactions, their role and the mechanisms in which they are involved, the identification of new diagnostic and therapeutic targets. The identification of protein biomarkers may be the basis for developing new methods of early diagnosis and treatment [1]. In general, an ideal biomarker should meet certain characteristics: be specific to a particular disease, be validated and confirmed as having specificity for that pathology, be able to early identify the disease, its testing to be easy and cheap as far as possible, reliable, and noninvasive [2, 3].

IntechOpen

Although important advances have been made in deciphering immune function, the understanding of this function dysregulation and the specific autoimmune response remains limited. The domain is complex and includes, besides the disturbance of immune system functioning, gene alterations that regulate and control the self-tolerance. In this chapter, we will describe the techniques of highlighting the proteomic biomarkers involved in the pathogenesis of immunogenetic diseases.

In the case of immunogenetic diseases, one of the tissues that are first tested for specific biomarkers is blood, namely, the serum, which contains approximately 60–80 mg/mL proteins, besides amino acids, lipids, salts, and carbohydrates [4]. Applying proteomic immunoassay techniques for the diagnosis of immunogenetic diseases may also predict the course of disease, or result in a personalized treatment for patients [5, 6].

Proteomic biomarkers are particularly useful for providing the information on cellular signaling pathways, bringing early disease data, monitoring treatment response or adverse effects. They can be monitored from body fluids other than blood, such as: urine, saliva, cerebrospinal fluid and from different tissues (biopsies) [7].

The necessity to analyze very small amounts of proteins present in biological samples [8], as well as the increase in the number of proteins requiring simultaneous, reliable, reproducible, and significant investigations led to the modernization of the existing techniques and to the appearance of some new methods of biomarker investigation and analysis. Immunohistochemistry, ELISA, and Western blotting are of the old methods that changed, adapted, modernized over time, but remained "on barricades" for protein biomarker investigation, especially in autoimmune disorders. Immunoassay methodologies are the most commonly used tools in protein research, using the properties of antibodies to bind different protein domains and to mark them. Next, the methods abovementioned are the other high sensitivity technics for validating proteomic biomarkers such as protein microarray, surface plasmon resonance, and Luminex multiplex assays. In recent years, many multiplexed immunodetection techniques have been developed to simultaneously investigate multiple proteins (from several tens to several hundreds), in the same sample, and which are in very low amounts (**Figure 1**).

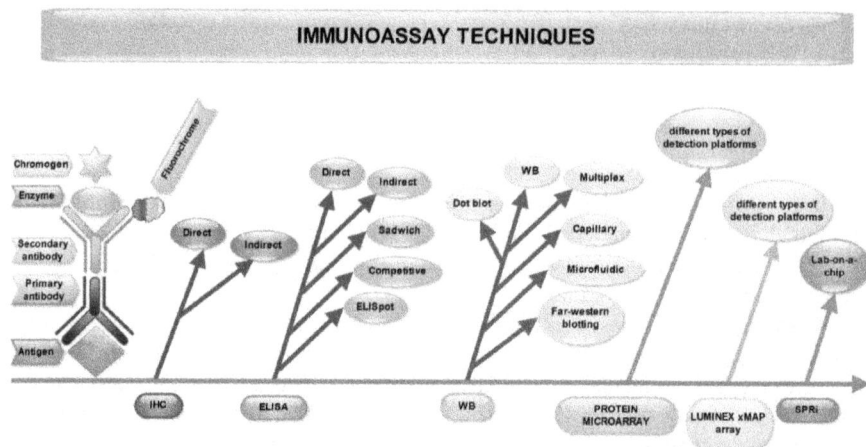

Figure 1.
The schematic representation of the immunoassay methods presented in this chapter, more or less in the order in which they appeared in time and how they evolved. These methods are based on the protein/antigen-antibody reaction that is shown on the left side—here is the indirect method: antigen → primary antibody → secondary antibody conjugated with a fluorochrome or an enzyme.

In many cases, the immunoassay techniques are used in conjunction for diagnostic, to confirm the presence of autoantibodies and then to characterize the expression of one or more specific biomarkers for a certain disease. More of this, these techniques can validate their mutual results.

2. Immunohistochemistry

The technique of immunohistochemistry (IHC) is a basic one, both in the anatomopathological diagnosis and in the research. It allows viewing of a protein of interest in a tissue section, specifying its location. This last aspect is very important and distinct IHC from other immunodetection techniques. The presence, reduction or the absence of the target protein allows a precise diagnosis or a personalized one. We do not intend to describe the technique itself, but we would like to mention it as the method of identifying immune antigens of interest, including immunogenetic diseases.

Based on the principle of the antigen-antibody reaction, this technique has undergone improvements over time. It started with a *direct IHC method*, the reaction antigen (target protein)-antibody, coupled with a fluorochrome. The first data on an attempt to use the direct IHC are from 1934 [9], but the use of fluorochrome for the first time was described in 1941 [10]. The introduction of an enzyme conjugated with an antibody and the visualization of the protein in light microscopy is due to Nakane and Pierce team [11]. The disadvantage of the IHC direct method is its low sensitivity.

Afterwards, an *IHC indirect method* was developed as follows: antigen-primary antibody, nonconjugated-secondary antibody (anti-primary antibody), conjugated with a fluorochrome or an enzyme, which convert a soluble substrate into an insoluble colored substrate [12, 13]. This method allowed the visual signal to be intensified.

The need to improve more the signal amplification has led to new changes. Thus the secondary antibody has been conjugated with other substances, such as biotin molecules, which in turn form complexes with streptavidin, forming a complex with an enzyme (e.g., horseradish peroxidase) [14]. More recently, an even more sensitive method was used in which a large number of secondary antibodies and enzymes are conjugated to a polymer chain (e.g., dextran) [15].

In the IHC technique, even *an array-like reaction* can be carried out on the same tissue section by targeting several proteins by using antibodies from different species (mouse, rabbit, goat, etc.), different enzymes coupled to the secondary antibody (e.g., horseradish peroxidase and alkaline phosphatase), different chromogens (e.g., 3,3′diaminobenzidine or 5-bromo-4-chloro-3-indolyl phosphate/nitro blue tetrazolium) or fluorochromes (e.g., FITC and rhodamine) with different colors.

Sometimes, especially when the protein of interest is low and the immunohistochemical signal is weak or with interruptions, a confirmation for protein expression by Western blotting is required. This confirmation is also required when we are not sure whether the antibody specifically binds to the protein of interest or if there is a nonspecific antibody labeling. The Western blot technique allows the identification of the protein as it is shown below.

3. Enzyme-linked immunosorbent assay (ELISA)

Old traditional ELISA technique was developed in 1971 by Engvall and Perlmann [16] and Van Weemen and Schuurs [17] and continues to be nowadays widely used as a routine diagnostic method allowing quantitation of a large variety of proteins [18]. The single-plex ELISA, the most utilized assay method performed in 96- or 384-well plates, has played a prominent role in the quantitative and qualitative identification of analytes.

Direct ELISA, the simplest type of ELISA, could accurately quantify a specific molecule with high sensitivity from a wide variety of samples, and it is faster [19]. But the signal is less amplified.

Indirect ELISA detection is a two-step ELISA which involves a primary antibody and a labeled secondary antibody [20]. This method presents a higher sensitivity and flexibility (different primary detection antibodies can be used with a single labeled secondary antibody). The disadvantage is the occurrence of nonspecific signals.

Beside direct and indirect detection models, two other ELISA methods appeared, to avoid false positive or false negative results, with a high specificity, suitable for complex samples, with more sensitivity and flexibility: *sandwich ELISA* (quantify antigens between the two layers of antibodies) [21] and *competitive ELISA* (based on a competitive binding process between the original antigen in the sample and the add-in antigen, the more antigen in the sample, the less labeled antigen is retained in the well and the weaker the signal) [22].

Another ELISA method is *ELISpot assay*, widely used to evaluate an immune response, for example, in allergies or in autoimmunity [23, 24]. This technique, performed on PVDF membranes, has advantages like specificity, sensitivity, and wide range of detection.

However, the use of ELISA for assessing multiple analytes might be time con- suming due to the large number of workflows occurring simultaneously. Moreover, ELISA is designed as a solid-state immunoassay, and the use of a planar matrix can restrict immunoassay capacity, sensitivity, and detection quality [25].

Conventional single-target assays ELISA and Western blot are suitable for bio- marker validation, but could be expensive, time consuming, and sample limiting. While most of the disease conditions may arise when only one single molecule is altered, more often it is the consequence of the interaction between several mol- ecules within the inflammation milieu; therefore, studying the diseases necessitates a comprehensive perspective.

ELISA on a chip. In order to improve the method, in terms of using smaller quan- tities of samples, shortening the reaction time, avoiding sophisticated reading equip- ment, and reducing costs, a group of researchers tried to miniaturize the ELIZA platform [26]. They developed an ELIZA lab-on-a-chip system (ELIZA-LOC), which allows the use of only 5 μl of sample on a miniaturized 96-well plate combined with a CCD camera [27]. This system combines three functional elements: (i) reagent load- ing fluidics, (ii) assay and detection well plate, and (iii) reagent removal fluidics. The description of LOM technology (laminated object manufacturing) to obtain this system using polymer sheets was made by Rasooly et al. [28].

Besides miniaturization, another novelty is the washing step that is integrated directly in ELISA plate. The authors state that using this technology, there is no need for a specialized laboratory to perform the ELIZA test.

4. Western blot

The Western blot (WB), also known as immunoblot, is an analytical and quantitative technique for identifying specific proteins in many biological samples, liquid or tissue/cellular homogenates [29]. The WB technique brings concrete and useful information that cannot be offered by other immunoassay methods. If the target protein, present in the sample, is altered qualitatively or quantitatively, the band thickness is changed compared to a control being downregulated or overexpressed. The WB results can also guide us to a genetic investigation in case of partial deletion or duplication in the protein gene [30]. In addition, the WB method allows a quick comparison of target protein expression in many patients in medical diagnosis.

The WB technique was invented by Harry Towbin and co-workers in 1979. They used the method to identify bacterial or chicken ribosomal proteins separated on polyacrylamide gels containing urea. They called this method "electrophoretic blotting technique" [31]. The WB name was given 2 years later by Neal Burnette, which also brought some improvements to this method, including the use of SDS-PAGE gels [32]. The name "Western" was inspired by the earlier name of other blotting methods, "Southern", named after the name of Edwin Southern, who published in 1975 a method for detecting specific DNA sequences [33], and "Northern" whose name was inspired by the name of the first blotting technique, "Southern", a RNA detection technique, developed in 1977 by Alwine et al. [34].

Over time, the method has improved and has become easier to achieve, with nearly all materials commercially available: transfer devices, antibodies, pre-casting gels, digital imaging devices, and so on. However, in the most part, as methodology, the technique proposed by the Towbin team remains valid after 38 years. Burnette, Stark, and Towbin said after many years that they were surprised by the success and longevity of the method [35].

In summary, the Western blot method is a way to identify a target protein from a biological sample, a mixture of proteins, running it on polyacrylamide gel. The proteins in the sample are separated by SDS-PAGE gel electrophoresis, depending on their molecular weight. Because the gel is hard to handle, being fragile, the proteins are transferred to a membrane, usually nitrocellulose or PVDF (polyvinylidene fluoride), that maintains the gel pattern as a copy [7]. The electrical current causes the transfer. For visualization of the protein of interest, the membrane is probed by a specific primary antibody, it binds the specific epitope of the protein, and it is labeled by addition of a secondary antibody recognizing the primary antibody conjugated with a detection reagent (fluorophore, enzyme, and radioisotope). The visualization is done colorimetric, by chemiluminescence, on X-ray film, or directly in the membrane with the aid of an imaging system.

In order to be able to reuse a WB membrane that has already been exposed to primary and secondary antibodies, it is necessary to wash it. This operation is called stripping. Only membranes that have been treated with ECL (enhanced *chemiluminescence kit*) for protein visualization by chemiluminescence can be reused. This method is useful when we want to investigate more proteins on the same blot, for example, a protein of interest and a loading control protein. It saves biological samples, time, and substances. For stripping, special buffers are using that can efficiently remove antibodies but do not remove too much amount of the proteins on the membrane.

The WB system size may vary, with electrophoresis/transfer tank, gels, and membrane: mini, midi, and large, depending on the investigated protein size and the time needed for separation. However, the vast majority of investigators use now the mini system, sometimes the midi one, because of the existence of gradient gels and more sophisticated devices (see below). Transfer systems were developed by few companies to allow proteins the migration from gel to the membrane in different ways, using varying amounts of buffers: wet, semidry, or dry systems. New digital technologies offer a good and rapid bands visualization, avoiding underexposure or overexposure, as in the case of X-ray film developing. The images can be stored in a computer database and can be analyzed with software that measures the optical density of the bands.

4.1 Other methods based on the Western blotting technique

4.1.1 Multiplex Western blot

In the last few years, it has become a necessity to analyze multiple target proteins at the same time, in order to compare the expression of proteins involved in a specific pathology. First Multiplex WB experiment (multiplex Western blot (MWB)) was optimized by Anderson and Davison [36] to study different muscle proteins involved in muscular dystrophies. This method allowed a simultaneously screening of multiple proteins with a different size on a pair of blots, using a cocktail of monoclonal antibodies which permitted the identification of primary deficient and second deficient proteins in several muscle pathologies, knowing that the primary reduction of a protein causes the secondary reduction of another protein. The use of a MWB allowed establishing a biomarker profile for each patient, providing valuable information for diagnosis as well as for phenotype-genotype correlations. The MWB method proposed by Anderson used a biphasic polyacrylamide gel (with different concentrations) system electrophoresis, which separated the proteins with different molecular weights: molecular mass more than 200 kDa in the upper part of the gel, with 5.5–4% polyacrylamide gradient, while proteins with molecular mass under 150 kDa are separated in the lower phase, 7% polyacrylamide gel.

Introduction of this technique has revolutionized the medical diagnosis and opened new perspectives in biomedical research. Simultaneous analysis of several proteins involved in different pathologies by MWB reduced the cost and time for analysis. By this method, it could be determined and compared proteins in the same sample as well as a secondary reduction of other proteins in a specific disease [37, 38].

4.1.2 Capillary electrophoresis and capillary Western blotting

By this method, the molecules are separated by the size inside a capillary filled with an electrolyte. The advantage of the method is that the separating sieve matrix can be automatically pumped in and out because it contains rather unknown polymers than the typical cross-linked polymers for the gels. The big difference between the classical method and this one is that many samples can be run over and over again in an automated manner that saves a lot of time [35].

Capillary electrophoresis (CE) needs a smaller amount of sample than SDS-PAGE and offers a better resolution of a protein size. Proteins travel down the capillaries and are spaced according to the size. When the individual proteins reach the end of the capillary, they drop on a blotting membrane that moves along the capillary opening. It has been shown that classical protein standards such as carbonic anhydrase and lysozyme can be separated within an hour using only a few nanoliters of the sample [39].

O'Neill et al. [40] have been able to capture the resolved proteins on the capillary wall by photochemically activated molecules. This method allowed immune complexes to be formed after electrophoresis, in the capillary. Chemiluminescence reagents flowed through the capillary, and the image was taken with a CCD camera [40].

4.1.3 Microfluidic Western blotting

This technology reduces much more the amount of the sample required for WB and also the length of the capillaries from centimeters to microns, using microfluidic channels. He and Herr, in 2009, developed an automated immunoblotting method using a single streamlined microfluidic assay. A glass microfluidic chip, which has integrated a PAGE electrophoresis with subsequent in situ immunoblotting, allowed a rapid protein separation, directed electrophoretic transfer of resolved proteins to an in-line blotting membrane, and a high-efficiency identification of proteins of interest using antibody-functionalized membranes [41, 42]. The system requires only 0.01–0.5 µg of protein.

4.1.4 Dot blot

It is a method very similar to WB, but the proteins are not separated by gel electrophoresis. The samples are applied in small dots directly on the membrane and then spotted through circular templates. After membrane drying, the antibodies are applied. The visualization of target protein is made like at WB, chemiluminescent or colorimetric. Dot blot is used to test the specificity of some antibodies, to test the antibody concentration used for WB, or to evaluate the presence of a target protein in the sample before WB.

4.1.5 Far-Western blotting

It is used to detect a protein-protein interaction *in vitro*. Instead of the primary antibody for detecting the protein of interest, this method uses a nonantibody protein that binds to the protein of interest. Far-Western blotting detects proteins on the basis of the presence or the absence of binding sites for the protein probe. This method is important in characterization of protein interactions in biological processes such as signal transductions [43], receptor-ligand interactions, or screen libraries for interacting proteins.

5. Protein microarray

Protein microarray analysis has an increasingly use both for research purposes as well as for various biomedical applications, *including the niches ones* like evaluating markers of apoptosis activated by various therapies such as photodynamic therapy (PDT), assessment of epigenetic milieu, or transcriptional activity in treated cells [44]. Thus, protein microarray is a proteomic tool that can deliver high-throughput data for revealing new therapeutic targets [45].

Protein microarray history has spanned the last two decades, the basic principle being identical with ELISA, but there are several advantages such as spotting in terms of miniaturization, multiplexing, and large data obtained in an ELISA equivalent time. Briefly, biological samples of interest (e.g., serum, plasma, etc.) are incubated on a slide containing immobilized antibodies, proteins, or peptides. An antigen-antibody reaction occurs between an analyte from the tested sample and the corresponding antibody from slide followed by the detection step through various methods (e.g., fluorescence-based detection). The slide is further scanned, followed by image acquisition, data processing, and analysis. There are several classifications of this technique, but it could fall into two main categories: direct phase (e.g., antibody-, protein-, peptide array) and reverse or indirect phase where sample of interest is spotted on a slide and the corresponding antibody is further added.

Among all these variants, the antibody array type is preferred in tumor research domain or in biomarkers discovery/quantification due to technique's high versatility and reproducibility [46]. The reverse phase array format could also be used for biomarker discovery because it is specificity but has the disadvantage of being more laborious.

It is worth to emphasize that protein microarray could be customized in terms of number and multiplicity of tested analytes one achieving new research and clinical benefits through this technology. Thus, although fundamental research purposes prevail when it comes to array platforms, there is also a recent increasing trend in clinical research, diagnostics, and even industry applications such as pharmacy or food. For instance, recent attempts are made in using array platform for autoimmune disease insights. Thus, novel antigen arrays have been developed in order to discover new autoantibody targets, providing analysis for hundreds of samples and of their reactivity pattern against thousands of antigens simultaneously [47].

Customizing an array in relation to clinical purpose confirms the flexibility of these platforms in assisting molecular management of the disease. A customized platform was designed in order to monitor severe acute respiratory syndrome (SARS) infection by screening hundreds of sera based on the reactivity against certain selected proteins from SARS coronavirus. Authors have reported that with this customized array, viral infection could be monitored for many months after infection [48]. This type of microarray platform has been further updated to a serological assay for the specific detection of IgM and IgG antibodies against the S1 receptor-binding subunit of the spike protein of emerging human coronavirus hCoV-EMC and SARS-CoV as antigens [49].

Protein microarray is a technology in continuous evolution offering multiple possibilities in updating other proteomic techniques. Therefore, the development of the "microwestern array" is a clear proof how traditional methods like Western blot can be linked to novel technology, thus significantly expanding the research technological arsenal [50].

Data generated by ELISA and WB require sometimes additional complementary proteomic methods to supplement and even support the scientific information. Such supportive task is often accomplished by protein microarrays providing important evidence on modulation of signaling networks and potential targets (or pathways); these factors or networks must first be identified, and array platforms allow exactly this development by exploring dozens of targets simultaneously within a single sample, providing lots of data which may be further investigated using traditional ELISA or WB techniques [51].

6. Luminex xMAP array

An important improvement in the biological assay field was made in the late 1990s when Luminex xMAP technology was launched. xMAP technology combines the principles of ELISA and flow cytometry, but goes beyond the limitations of solid-phase reaction kinetics and is suitable for high throughput, multiplex, and simultaneous detection of different biomarkers within a very small volume sample. Bringing together advanced fluidics, optics, and digital signal processing with proprietary microspheres, xMAP technology became one of the fastest growing multiplex technologies. Featuring a flexible open-architecture design, xMAP technology enables the configuration of various assays, quickly, cost effectively, and accurately, useful in clinical and research laboratories [52].

A key component of Luminex xMAP technology is represented by proprietary color-code polystyrene microspheres (beads) internally dyed with precise concentrations of two or three spectrally distinct fluorochromes. Through precise concentrations of these specific dyes, up to 500 distinctly bead sets can be developed, with a different spectral signature.

Based on fluorescent reporter signals, high-speed digital-signal processors identify each individual microsphere and quantify the result of every bioassay. The capability of adding multiple conjugated beads to each sample results in the ability to obtain multiple results from each sample [53].

There are different types of advanced detection platforms (as depicted in **Table 1**), and therefore, various biomarker panels could be analyzed. Accordingly, validation of novel biomarkers into multiplex immunoassay panels confers an attractive prospect of simultaneous measurement of multiple analytes in a single patient sample, enabling progres-sion monitoring and outcome prediction, even detecting major diseases in its earliest stages [54].

Technique	Advantages	Disadvantages	Use
IHC	Qualitative Fast Easy to detect Relatively inexpensive	Medium specificity Possible cross reactivity	Routine diagnstic tool Shows the localisation of antigen
ELISA	Quantitative High sensitivity Medium specificity Higher throughput than Western blot Automation potential	One protein/analyte at a time False positive results Labor intensive/time consuming/high reagent use Costly setup for automation	To quantify a single protein Confirmation of other screening method/validation
Western blot	High specificity High sensitivity Quantitative Automation potential	One or a small number of proteins/analytes at a time Labor intensive/time consuming for the classical method. Resolved by the new equipments Qualitative, quantitative, especially with the newest equipments Difficult to transfer large or hydrophobic proteins—false negative results Difficult to automate—for the classical method. Resolved by the new equipments	To identify the presence of a small number of proteins in the same sample (multiplex WB) or the presence of protein-protein interactions (Far-WB) Confirmation of other screening method/antibodies validation
Bead-based array (e.g., Luminex® technology)	High sensitivity High throughput and speed Multiplex and customizable panels of analytes Open-architecture design Low time, labor, and reagent use over traditional methods Versatility Flexibility	High cost for a specialized equipment and a validated antibody pair	To quantify (quantitative) multiple proteins/panels of analytes, in the same well from a small amount of sample Clinical implementation—available IVD kits
Protein microarray	High sensitivity Medium specificity Highest throughput Low time and reagent use	High cost for a specialized equipment and a validated antibody pair	To screen for changes across a large number of proteins, in the same well from a small amount of sample

Technique	Advantages	Disadvantages	Use
SPRi	Very high sensitivity Label-free Real time method High throughput and speed Multiplex and customizable panels of analytes Open-architecture design Low time, labor, and reagent use over traditional methods Low time and reagent use Biochip reusable	High cost for a specialized equipment Suitable for liquid biological probes	To screen and quantify (quantitative) multiple protein interactions (and not only)/ panels of analytes, from the same sample Clinical implementation

Table 1.
Advantages and disadvantages of immunoassay methods presented in this chapter: IHC, ELISA, Western blot, bead-based array—Luminex technology, and chip-based array—protein microarray, SPRi.

Some of our studies illustrate significant dysregulation in circulating levels of cytokines and angiogenic factors in brain tumors, with over threefold upregulation of IL-6, IL-1 beta, TNF-alpha, and IL-10 and up to twofold upregulation of VEGF, FGF-2, IL-8, IL-2, and GM-CSF, with implications in tumor progression and aggressiveness, and also involved in disease-associated pain [55, 56].

Currently, Western blot is used to validate/confirm the identified biomarkers, and association between the xMAP technology and the Western blot was remarked in many studies. Interestingly, one of them emphasized the improvement in diagnostic sensitivity of HIV infection in early stages using xMAP technology, increasing the chances of an early accurate diagnosis. Thus, it was observed a superior sensitivity of Luminex xMAP compared with Western blot. Out of 87 confirmed HIV positive cases, Western blot confirmed 74.7% sensitivity, while Luminex xMAP identified 82.8% sensitivity ($p < 0.05$) [57]. Further advancements will be needed for a successful validation of current discoveries, and sustained efforts are necessary to expand the translation into clinical applications toward personalized medicine [58].

7. Surface plasmon resonance imaging, lab-on-a-chip

Since our goal is not describing surface plasmon resonance imaging (SPRi) methodology, we will not insist very much on the description of the technique. We will make a brief description of the principle on which SPRi is based.

The first SPR immunoassay was proposed by the team Liedberg, Nylander, and Lundström, in 1983 [59]. The SPR immunoassay method is label-free (unlike ELISA); no label molecule is required for analyte detection [60]. Moreover, the measurement is done in real time, which allows monitoring of the individual steps of this technology. SPRi is currently one of the most sensible platforms for studying a wide variety of interaction affinities [61, 62], involving nucleic acid sequences [63–65], peptides [66], proteins [67, 68], and carbohydrates [69]. It is possible to monitor hundreds of molecular interactions simultaneously.

The composition of a biochip consists essentially of a glass prism, coated with a thin gold film and a pre-functionalized surface chemistry. The sample to be analyzed is injected over the biochip, and the detection of a specific molecule can be performed by immobilizing a binding partner on the biochip. SPRi makes a nonlabeling and a real-time detection of biomarkers [70].

The SPRi platform allows the quantitative detection of multiple simultaneous multiplex interactions, and many studies are based on this application for screening a variety of analytes in different array types. The main advantage of using SPRi in immunodiagnostics is the possibility of monitoring the antigen-antibody reaction in real-time, estimating kinetics, how quickly it occurs and how durable it is. In addition, it does not require any labels.

In comparison to ELISA and Western Blot, SPRi has the advantage of investigating a large number of different analytes from the same sample (several hundred different spots can be placed on a biochip), and after washing the biochip, it is possible to immediately analyze another sample. SPRi takes less time than other methods. The disadvantage of SPRi would be that only liquid biological samples (blood, urine, cerebrospinal fluid, and cell culture medium) can be analyzed, and it does not analyze biological samples from different tissues/tissue lysates. SPRi is very effective when there are many samples and many different interactions to analyze, but for a small number of samples or to demonstrate only one type of interaction between two proteins, for example, WB is more efficient.

As a conclusion regarding the technologies presented in this chapter, we show **Table 1** with the advantages and disadvantages of each method.

8. Immunoassay methods in immunogenetic disease diagnostic

Indirect immunofluorescence (IIF) for autoantibody analysis is one of the routine diagnostic methods. Different tissue sections or human tumor cell lines—HEp-2— are used as the source of antigen over which the serum of patients with specific autoantibodies is applied [71].

The antinuclear antibody (ANA) test is such a standard screening assay. The American College of Rheumatology declared HEp-2 IIF as the preferred method for ANA screening [72]. The large amount of ANAs can indicate an autoimmune disease, including systemic lupus erythematosus, Sjogren's syndrome, scleroderma, rheumatoid arthritis, idiopathic inflammatory myopathy, and others.

One of the immunohistochemistry method applications in autoimmune disease diagnosis is the detection of the presence of MHC I and, more recently, of MHC II in skeletal muscle of patients with idiopathic inflammatory myopathies (IIMs). It is a group of autoimmune systemic diseases, of which the most common forms are dermatomyositis, polymyositis, and inclusion body myositis. The study of muscle biopsy makes the difference in diagnosis between subtypes, but also among other types of myopathies and IIMs. In addition to other pathological features, the presence of MHC I and MHC II in sarcolemma gives the certainty of diagnosis, as long as they are not present in normal muscles [73–76]. Their overexpression in IIMs is induced by cytokines, including interferon and tumor necrosis factor alpha (TNF alpha) [77]. A study of 120 muscle biopsies from patients with different forms of IIMs showed a presence of MHC I in all biopsies and MHC II in 93% of them [76].

The MHC I expression appears early and precedes the lymphocyte infiltrate [78], persisting in late disease, and it is not attenuated by immunosuppressive treatment [79–81].

MHC II expression on antigen presenting cells activates T-helper cells and initiates an immune response without knowing the mechanism by which MHC II alleles mediate susceptibility to a given autoimmune disease [82].

From our experience in IIM cases where the IHC is not conclusive, a WB verification or validation is of great help in highlighting MHC I and II bands at their specific molecular weight.

From the more recent studies, we mention that the anti-signal recognition particle antibodies in the serum of IIM patients have diagnostic and prognostic value especially in the forms of immune-mediated necrotizing myopathy [83]. The authors draw attention to a mandatory IIF test along with the dot immunoassay to avoid false positive results from the latter method in pathologies not associated with IIM. The results sometimes depend on the nature of the antigen used in the technique and can be denatured.

ELISA is used as a diagnostic tool in autoimmune diseases, for evaluation of serum autoantibodies. Antinuclear antibodies (ANAs) directed against a variety of nuclear and cytoplasmic antigens are found with a high frequency in many systemic autoimmune disorders like systemic lupus erythematosus, scleroderma, Sjogren's syndrome, myositis, etc. *ANA-HEp-2 Screen ELISA* is an immunoassay method for the qualitative combined detection of IgG antibodies against human serum HEp-2 cells. Each well is coated with Hep-2 cellular lysate. The test detects in a well plate total ANAs against double stranded DNA, histone, SS-A (Ro), SS-B (La), Sm, snRNP/Sm, Scl-70, PM-Scl, Jo-1, and centromeric antigens.

HEp-2 cells allow the recognition of over 30 nuclear and cytoplasmic patterns that are given upwards of 50 different autoantibodies [84, 85]. The specificity of the test is closely related to the quality of the antigens used [86]. It is one of the most common methods of diagnosis in organ-specific autoimmune diseases, such as Grave's disease, primary biliary cirrhosis, insulin-dependent diabetes mellitus or systemic autoimmune disorders affecting different organs, such as systemic sclerosis, Sjogren's syndrome, and mixed connective tissue disease rheumatoid arthritis [87, 88].

From recent research studies [89], we want to mention cortactin antibodies as new biomarkers in double seronegative myasthenia gravis (myasthenia gravis form dSNMG). ELISA tests validated by WB have demonstrated that the presence of cortactin autoantibodies is a biomarker to be taken into account, suggesting that the disease will be ocular or mild generalized and could be done routinely in the future.

Another work on rheumatoid arthritis shows that, apart from the autoantibody system that recognizes citrullinated proteins, the identification of another antibody system against carbamylated proteins has an important early diagnostic value, predicting a more severe course of disease [90]. The ELISA method used in this study could become routine for serum testing of patients with rheumatoid arthritis.

Western blot. To highlight the importance of WB technique in clinical diagnosis, we give some eloquent examples below. The WB method has been used in many studies, along with immunoprecipitation, ELISA, and flow cytometry, to demonstrate the quantitative or qualitative modification of proteins of interest in autoimmune diseases in order to find new biomarkers or therapeutic targets. WB has proven to be a good tool for serological tests.

Line-blot immunoassay is a Western blotting method that uses recombinant antigens immobilized on straight lines on a nylon strip. They are incubated with patient serum containing autoantibodies. They bind to the antigens present on the strip and are viewed colorimetrically. Interpretation of the results is done by comparing the color intensity of strips with the color of strips of a positive standard. There are some studies that have shown the utility of this method in the detection of autoantibodies present in serum but which could not be identified by IIF, for example, anti-SS-A/Ro in Sjogren's syndrome [91, 92].

Haroon et al. have demonstrated using the WB method that there is an interaction between endoplasmic reticulum aminopeptidase 1 (ERAP1) with human leucocyte antigen (HLA)-B *27 in ankylosing spondylitis [93], and that the HLA-B27 molecules could alter the ERAP1 level. The functional interaction between ERAP1-peptide and HLA-B27 could thus be the missing link in the pathogenesis of ankylosing spondylitis.

Stagakis et al. studied whether anti-TNF therapy improves insulin resistance in rheumatoid arthritis [94]. Western blot was used to analyze the proteins p-Ser^{312} IRS-1 and p-AKT from peripheral blood mononuclear cell lysates. It has been established that anti-TNF alpha therapy has a positive effect, improving insulin sensitivity and reversing the defects in signaling insulin cascade in this disease.

Tsui et al. have conducted a study of the serum levels of noggin (NOG) and sclerostin (SOST) in patients with ankylosing spondylitis, more specifically, on the immune response to these two molecules [95]. The WB method was used to quantify the relative amounts of NOG/SOST-IgG immune complexes. An increased level of NOG/SOST-IgG immune complexes was found in patients with this pathology.

Rizzo et al. [96] showed that the dimeric form of the HLA-G molecule is associated with the response to methotrexate treatment in patients with early rheumatoid arthritis. HLA-G dimeric and monomeric forms have been highlighted by WB. The presence of dimeric form in plasma prior to methotrexate therapy could be a biomarker for the patient's response to treatment.

Protein microarray. Antibody microarrays could provide a real-time vision of biological processes, such proteomic instrument being used in clinic to analyze serum and plasma in several pathologies including autoimmune disorders. One of the autoimmune diseases approached through protein array is *systemic lupus erythematosus* (SLE) where SLE clinical heterogeneity and the absence of robust biomarkers to evaluate the disease states and differentiate from other autoimmune conditions are yet to be resolved [97]. Thus, using an antibody-based leukocyte-capture microarray, mononuclear cells isolated from peripheral blood of 60 SLE patients were processed for obtaining proteomic patterns to distinguish SLE from healthy subjects. With this array platform, it was improved the conventional SLE diagnostics and disease states elucidation [98]. Moreover, an "in-house" antibody microarray comprising 135 human recombinant single-chain fragment variables aiming various immune proteins were used to examine *systemic sclerosis* (SSc) and SLE patients. This tailored array identified a significant number of differentially expressed proteins that delineate SLE from systemic sclerosis, thus surpassing disease classification through conventional clinical parameters, including, ANA, anti-DNA, SLEDAI-2 k, C1q, C3, C4, and CRP [99].

Another challenging field for protein array is related to *rheumatoid arthritis* (RA) as it could detect biomarkers specific for arthritis and not for autoimmune diseases in general [100]. Some research groups have started to develop different antigen arrays for differential diagnosis and even RA molecular classifying. Panels of proteins were detected, among these three proteins, namely, WIBG, GABARALP2, and ZNF706, were suggested as potential specific markers for RA early stages [101]. Hence, protein arrays bring valuable data to immune-disease background allowing exploration of numerous samples in parallel and thousands of targets.

Antibodies against ion channels, receptors, synaptic proteins, etc. confirm protein microarrays as a future potential tool in routine diagnosis [102]. Whatever commercially available or customized platforms, antibody arrays start to emerge in clinic by designing *omics* disease signatures helping the disease management.

The protein microarray was used in a study of *pemphigus vulgaris*, an autoimmune skin disease, to identify the entire set of antibodies, bringing extra data about the complex relationship between genetics and disease development [103]. The results were correlated with those obtained by the ELISA and proved to be compatible. The main targets for autoantibodies are desmoglein-3 and 1, but the study showed that there are autoantibodies that are not directed to desmoglein at a significant number of patients.

A study regarding *ankylosing spondylitis* using the protein microarray, confirmed by ELISA, to characterize anti-ankylosing spondylitis autoantibodies, showed that anti-protein phosphatase 1A (PPM1A) autoantibodies are present in the serum of the patients and that they could serve not only as biomarkers for diagnosis, disease severity, and response to anti-TNF therapy, but also as a therapeutic target [104].

Luminex xMAP technology has developed as an alternative to planar microarray methods. Bead-based immunoassays are one of them. The determinations by this method and by ELISA of anti-thyroid peroxidase and anti-thyroglobulin antibodies in autoimmune diseases have been shown to be compatibles [105].

There is a commercially available kit for ANA detection, which is low cost and saves time. Antigens corresponding to autoantibodies are linked to polystyrene microspheres labeled internally with different amounts of two different fluoro-chromes, resulting in 100 different color spectra. Each microbead carries an antigen specific for a single antibody [106].

Good results were obtained in assessing a number of antinuclear autoantibodies as: dsDNA, Sm and Sm/RNP (in systemic lupus erythematosus), SS-A/Ro and SS-B/La (in Sjogren's syndrome), Jo-1 (myositis), ribosome (systemic lupus erythematosus), and centromere (systemic sclerosis) [107].

One of the problems with this technology could be the lack of a true quantitative calibration due to the difference in affinity of the antibodies for the antigen [108]. Some authors argue that it is also necessary to validate the results by other immuno-assay methods [106], while others claim that the accuracy of the technique is similar to that observed by ELISA [109, 110].

There are studies in which the Luminex methodology is used for the analysis of serum biomarkers in various autoimmune diseases. Thus, in an article on ankylos-ing spondylitis, certain cytokines as hepatocyte growth factor (HGF), CXCL8, and matrix metalloproteinases (MMP-8 and MMP-9) identified from a large number of biomarkers by Luminex could be diagnostic targets, their serum levels being increased in this disease [111].

In other chapter regarding ankylosing spondylitis, Luminex bead-based technology was used for serum cytokines analysis, and the conclusion was that the utilization of TNF alpha inhibitors decreases the number of T cells producing proinflammatory cytokines [112].

Mou et al. showed, using Luminex technology in combination with PCR, that in ankylosing spondylitis patients from Southern China with HLA-B27 in their serum, HLA-B2704 subtype predominates. And the HLA-B2715 subtype may have a disease prognostic value, early onset being related to this subtype [113].

Surface plasmon resonance imaging. Despite its great sensitivity, this technology is relatively little used to determine the concentration of some analytes. Improving signal amplification methods is one of the research goals in this technique.

In some autoimmune diseases, such as rheumatoid arthritis (RA), psoriatic arthritis, systemic lupus erythematosus, or Sjogren's syndrome, autoantibod-ies attack citrullinated proteins, and the presence of anti-citrullinated proteins, antibodies is a standard test in these cases. The use of SPRi for monitoring autoanti-bodies that bind to different citrullinated targets was first described by Lokate et al. SPRi has shown its ability to detect the interaction between citrullinated peptides and serum autoantibodies in RA patients in one step [114].

SPRi microarray technique was also used in a more recent research to identify autoantibodies against citrullinated protein (ACPA) profiles in patients with early onset rheumatoid arthritis. The authors made a comparative study using citrullinated and noncitrullinated peptides [115]. The study showed that SPRi is a suitable methodology for detecting ACPAs in the serum of patients with this pathology.

A subsequent study was also revealed by SPRi, the presence of citrullinated B-cell epitopes in fibrinogen [116].

A research team [117] showed the use of SPRi and gold particles to amplify the signal for the detection of inflammation biomarker TNF-alpha in serum. Also, the use of a specific buffer solution for sample dilution was utilized to reduce the nonspecific binding in real samples. Thus, a low limit of detection, as well as a good reproducibility and the longevity of chips, is a good motivation to use this immunoassay method to detect biomarkers that are in low concentrations in biological samples.

Buhl et al. reported in a research paper the use of SPRi technology for the anti-dsDNA detection in systemic lupus erythematosus [118].

9. Conclusions

Immunoassay methods have many advantages but some limitations too. Their importance in identifying different biomarkers for diagnosis or personalized therapy is essential. That is why they have diversified so much, in order to be able to answer all the challenges. Additionally, these methods and technologies have also specialized in an advanced degree, so that they can detect smaller amounts of molecules with as high a precision as possible in a shorter time. The antigen-antibody response gives them great sensitivity. The development of more advanced equipment leads to the automation of these methods and to a greater efficiency, with applicability in diagnosis and therapeutic monitoring, in discovery of new biomarkers and even in pharmacology.

In order to be used for diagnosis in different laboratories, these methods and kits should be standardized. The problems to be posed are: the clinical manifestation of the disease in different individuals, the source of the antigen, the specificity and sensitivity of the autoantibodies for different antigens, the reproducibility of the assay, and the precision and the accuracy of the method [91, 119, 120].

Some studies show a good correlation between IIF and ELISA methods [84, 121, 122], and others, on the contrary, show different results between these methods [71, 123].

Multiplex technologies are gaining more and more followers in recent years by allowing simultaneous analysis of a multitude of analysts, saving time and costs. However, there are studies showing that compared to the old methods, some false negative or false positive results are obtained [124–128]. Cross reactivities may also occur [129].

Assay kits produced by different manufacturers can show variable results also. More than this, the methodology used by each laboratory can lead to different results, even by using the same kit. International standardization is required. A collaboration between an international body and organizations responsible for quality of assessment of assays is desirable, so that a collaboration among clinicians, diagnostic laboratories, and manufacturers to be established.

Acknowledgements

All authors contributed equally to this work. Partially supported from Project ID: SMIS CSNR 1882/49159 (CAMED), PN-III-P1-1.2-PCCDI-2017-0341 (PATHDERM), PN-III-P1-1.2-PCCDI-2017-0782 (REGMED), PN 16.22.02.04/2016, PN 16.22.02.05/2016, PN 18.21.02.02/2018, and PN 18.21.01.06/2018.

Author details

Emilia Manole[1,2*], Alexandra E. Bastian[3,4], Ionela D. Popescu[1],
Carolina Constantin[1,2,5], Simona Mihai[1], Gisela F. Gaina[1,5], Elena Codrici[1]
and Monica T. Neagu[1,2,5]

1 National Institute of Pathology "Victor Babes", Bucharest, Romania

2 Colentina Clinical Hospital, Research Centre, Bucharest, Romania

3 Pathology Department, Colentina Clinical Hospital, Bucharest, Romania

4 University of Medicine "Carol Davila", Bucharest, Romania

5 Faculty of Biology, University of Bucharest, Bucharest, Romania

*Address all correspondence to: emilia_manole@yahoo.com

IntechOpen

© 2018 The Author(s). Licensee IntechOpen. This chapter is distributed under the terms of the Creative Commons Attribution License (http://creativecommons.org/licenses/by/3.0), which permits unrestricted use, distribution, and reproduction in any medium, provided the original work is properly cited. (cc) BY

References

[1] Hanash SM. Biomedical applications of two-dimensional electrophoresis using immobilized pH gradients: Current status. Electrophoresis. 2000;**21**:1202-1209

[2] National Institute of Aging Working group AB. Consensus report of the Working Group on: "Molecular and Biochemical Markers of Alzheimer's disease". Neurobiology of Aging. 1998;**19**(2):109-116

[3] Gao J, Garulacan LA, Storm SM, Opiteck GJ, Dubaquie Y, Hefta SA, et al. Biomarker discovery in biological fluids. Methods. 2005;**35**(3):291-302

[4] Burtis CA, Ashwood EA, editors. Tietz Fundamentals of Clinical Chemistry. 5th ed. 2001

[5] Robinson WH, Steinman L, Utz PJ. Proteomics technologies for the study of autoimmune disease. Arthritis & Rheumatism. 2002;**46**(4):885-893

[6] Hueber W, Robinson WH. Proteomic biomarkers for autoimmune disease. Proteomics. 2006;**6**(14):4100-4105

[7] Kurien BT, Scofield RH. Western blotting. Methods. 2006;**38**(4):283-293

[8] Coorssen JR, Blank PS, Albertorio F, Bezrukov L, Kolosova I, Backlund PS Jr, et al. Quantitative femto- to attomole immunodetection of regulated secretory vesicle proteins critical to exocytosis. Analytical Biochemistry. 2002;**307**(1):54-62

[9] Marrack J. Nature of antibodies. Nature. 1934;**133**:292-293

[10] Coons AH, Creech HJ, Jones RN. Immunological properties of an antibody containing a fluorescence group. Proceedings of the Society for Experimental Biology and Medicine. 1941;**47**(2):200-202

[11] Nakane PK, Pierce GB Jr. Enzyme-labeled antibodies: Preparation and application for the localization of antigens. Journal of Histochemistry and Cytochemistry. 1966;**14**(12):929-931

[12] Sternberger LA, Hardy PH Jr, Cuculis JJ, Meyer HG. The unlabeled antibody enzyme method of immunohistochemistry: Preparation and properties of soluble antigen-antibody complex (horseradish peroxidase-antihorseradish peroxidase) and its use in identification of spirochetes. Journal of Histochemistry and Cytochemistry. 1970;**18**(5):315-333

[13] Mason DY, Sammons R. Alkaline phosphatase and peroxidase for double immunoenzymatic labelling of cellular constituents. Journal of Clinical Pathology. 1978;**31**(5):454-460

[14] Hsu SM, Raine L. Protein A, avidin, and biotin in immunohistochemistry. Journal of Histochemistry and Cytochemistry. 1981;**29**(11):1349-1353

[15] Ramos-Vara JA, Miller MA. Comparison of two polymer-based immunohistochemical detection systems: ENVISION+ and ImmPRESS. Journal of Microscopy. 2006;**224**(Pt 2):135-139

[16] Engvall E, Perlmann P. Enzyme-linked immunosorbent assay (ELISA). Quantitative assay of immunoglobulin G. Immunochemistry. 1971;**8**(9):871-874

[17] Van Weemen BK, Schuurs AH. Immunoassay using antigen-enzyme conjugates. FEBS Letters. 1971;**15**(3):232-236

[18] Bilan R, Ametzazurra A, Brazhnik K, Escorza S, Fernandez D, Uribarri M, et al. Quantum-dot-based suspension microarray for multiplex detection of lung cancer markers: Preclinical

validation and comparison with the Luminex xMAP system. Scientific Reports. 2017;7:44668

[19] Engvall E. The ELISA, enzyme-linked immunosorbent assay. Clinical Chemistry. 2010;56:319-320

[20] Lindström P, Wager O. IgG autoantibody to human serum albumin studied by the ELISA-technique. Scandinavian Journal of Immunology. 1978;7(5):419-425

[21] Kato K, Hamaguchi Y, Okawa S, Ishikawa E, Kobayashi K. Use of rabbit antibody IgG bound onto plain and aminoalkylsilyl glass surface for the enzyme-linked sandwich immunoassay. Journal of Biochemistry. 1977;82(1):261-266

[22] Yorde DE, Sasse EA, Wang TY, Hussa RO, Garancis JC. Competitive enzyme-liked immunoassay with use of soluble enzyme/antibody immune complexes for labeling. I. Measurement of human choriogonadotropin. Clinical Chemistry. 1976;22(8):1372-1377

[23] Czerkinsky CC, Nilsson LA, Nygren H, Ouchterlony O, Tarkowski A. A solid-phase enzyme-linked immuno-spot (ELISPOT) assay for enumeration of specific antibody-secreting cells. Journal of Immunological Methods. 1983;65(1-2):109-121

[24] Franci C, Ingles J, Castro R, Vidal J. Further studies on the ELISA-spot technique. Its application to particulate antigens and potential improvement in sensitivity. Journal of Immunological Methods. 1986;88(2):225-232

[25] Liotta LA, Espina V, Mehta AI, Calvert V, Rosenblatt K, Geho D, et al. Protein microarrays: Meeting analytical challenges for clinical applications. Cancer Cell. 2003;3(4):317-325

[26] Sapsford KE, Francis J, Sun S, Kostov Y, Rasooly A. Miniaturized

96-well ELISA chips for staphylococcal enterotoxin B detection using portable colorimetric detector. Analytical and Bioanalytical Chemistry. 2009;394(2):499-505

[27] Sun S, Yang M, Kostov Y, Rasooly A. ELISA-LOC: Lab-on-a-chip for enzyme-linked immunodetection. Lab on a Chip. 2010;10(16):2093-2100

[28] Rasooly A, Bruck HA, Kostov Y. An ELISA Lab-on-a-chip (ELISA-LOC). Methods in Molecular Biology. 2013;949:451-471

[29] Ghosh R, Gilda JE, Gomes AV. The necessity of and strategies for improving confidence in the accuracy of western blots. Expert Review of Proteomics. 2014:1-12

[30] Barresi R. From proteins to genes: Immunoanalysis in the diagnosis of muscular dystrophies. Skeletal Muscle. 2011;1(1):24

[31] Towbin H, Staehelin T, Gordon J. Electrophoretic transfer of proteins from polyacrylamide gels to nitrocellulose sheets: Procedure and some applications. Proceedings of the National Academy of Sciences of the United States of America. 1979;76(9):4350-4354

[32] Burnette WN. "Western blotting": Electrophoretic transfer of proteins from sodium dodecyl sulfate-polyacrylamide gels to unmodified nitrocellulose and radiographic detection with antibody and radioiodinated protein A. Analytical Biochemistry. 1981;112(2):195-203

[33] Southern EM. Detection of specific sequences among DNA fragments separated by gel electrophoresis. Journal of Molecular Biology. 1975;98(3):503-517

[34] Alwine JC, Kemp DJ, Stark GR. Method for detection of specific

RNAs in agarose gels by transfer to diazobenzyloxymethyl-paper and hybridization with DNA probes. Proceedings of the National Academy of Sciences of the United States of America. 1977;**74**(12):5350-5354

[35] Mukhopadhyay R. Revamping the Western blot. ASBMB Today. 2012:14-16

[36] Anderson LV, Davison K. Multiplex western blotting system for the analysis of muscular dystrophy proteins. The American Journal of Pathology. 1999;**154**(4):1017-1022

[37] Gaina G, Manole E, Bordea C, Ionica E. Analysis of muscle Calpain-3 in LGMD 2A. Jurnal Studia Universitatis "Vasile Goldis" Arad. Seria Stiintele Vietii (Life Sciences Series). 2008;**18**:181-185

[38] Gaina G, Manole E, Matanie C, Mihalcea A, Ionica E. Muscular dystrophies proteins evaluation by western blott and immunofluorescence. Romanian Biotechnological Letters. 2008;**13**(3):3729-3736

[39] Anderson GJ, Cipolla CM, Kennedy RT. Western blotting using capillary electrophoresis. Analytical Chemistry. 2011;**83**:1350-1355

[40] O'Neill RA, Bhamidipati A, Bi X, Deb-Basu D, Cahill L, Ferrante J, et al. Isoelectric focusing technology quantifies protein signaling in 25 cells. PNAS. 2006;**103**(44):16153-16158

[41] He M, Herr AE. Microfluidic polyacrylamide gel electrophoresis with in situ immunoblotting for native protein analysis. Analytical Chemistry. 2009;**81**:8177-8184

[42] He M, Herr AE. Polyacrylamide gel photopatterning enables automated protein immunoblotting in a two-dimensional microdevice. Journal of the American Chemical Society. 2010;**132**:2512-2513

[43] Machida K, Mayer BJ. Detection of protein-protein interactions by far-western blotting. In: Kurien BT, Scofield RH, editors. Protein Blotting and Detection Methods in Molecular Biology (Methods and Protocols). Totowa, NJ: Humana Press; 2009

[44] Demyanenko SV, Uzdensky AB, Sharifulina SA, Lapteva TO, Polyakova LP. PDT-induced epigenetic changes in the mouse cerebral cortex: A protein microarray study. Biochimica et Biophysica Acta. 2014;**1840**(1):262-270

[45] Matei C, Tampa M, Caruntu C, Ion RM, Georgescu SR, Dumitrascu GR, et al. Protein microarray for complex apoptosis monitoring of dysplastic oral keratinocytes in experimental photodynamic therapy. Biological Research. 2014;**47**:33

[46] Wilson JJ, Burgess R, Mao YQ, Luo S, Tang H, Jones VS, et al. Antibody arrays in biomarker discovery. Advances in Clinical Chemistry. 2015;**69**:255-324

[47] Ayoglu B, Schwenk JM, Nilsson P. Antigen arrays for profiling autoantibody repertoires. Bioanalysis. 2016;**8**(10):1105-1126

[48] Zhu H, Hu S, Jona G, Zhu X, Kreiswirth N, Willey BM, et al. Severe acute respiratory syndrome diagnostics using a coronavirus protein microarray. Proceedings of the National Academy of Sciences of the United States of America. 2006;**103**(11):4011-4016

[49] Reusken C, Mou H, Godeke GJ, van der Hoek L, Meyer B, Muller MA, et al. Specific serology for emerging human coronaviruses by protein microarray. Eurosurveillance: Bulletin Europeen sur les Maladies Transmissibles = European Communicable Disease Bulletin. 2013;**18**(14):20441

[50] Mann M. Can proteomics retire the western blot? Journal of Proteome Research. 2008;**7**(8):3065

[51] Bass JJ, Wilkinson DJ, Rankin D, Phillips BE, Szewczyk NJ, Smith K, et al. An overview of technical considerations for Western blotting applications to physiological research. Scandinavian Journal of Medicine and Science in Sports. 2017;**27**(1):4-25

[52] http://info.luminexcorp.com/en-us/research/download-the-xmap-cookbook

[53] http://core.phmtox.msu.edu/Scheduling/ItemDocs/65/LuminexUserManual.pdf

[54] Tighe PJ, Ryder RR, Todd I, Fairclough LC. ELISA in the multiplex era: Potentials and pitfalls. Proteomics—Clinical Applications. 2015;**9**(3-4):406-422

[55] Albulescu R, Codrici E, Popescu ID, Mihai S, Necula LG, Petrescu D, et al. Cytokine patterns in brain tumour progression. Mediators of Inflammation. 2013;**2013**:979748

[56] Tanase C, Albulescu R, Codrici E, Popescu ID, Mihai S, Enciu AM, et al. Circulating biomarker panels for targeted therapy in brain tumors. Future Oncology. 2015;**11**(3):511-524

[57] Kong W, Li Y, Cheng S, Yan C, An S, Dong Z, et al. Luminex xMAP combined with western blot improves HIV diagnostic sensitivity. Journal of Virological Methods. 2016;**227**:1-5

[58] Krochmal M, Schanstra JP, Mischak H. Urinary peptidomics in kidney disease and drug research. Expert Opinion on Drug Discovery. 2017:1-10

[59] Ingemar LBNCL. Surface plasmon resonance for gas detection and biosensing. Sensors and Actuators. 1983;**4**:299-304

[60] Rich RL, Myszka DG. Higher-throughput, label-free, real-time molecular interaction analysis.

Analytical Biochemistry. 2007;**361**(1):1-6

[61] Paul S, Vadgama P, Ray AK. Surface plasmon resonance imaging for biosensing. IET Nanobiotechnology. 2009;**3**(3):71-80

[62] Scarano S, Mascini M, Turner AP, Minunni M. Surface plasmon resonance imaging for affinity-based biosensors. Biosensors and Bioelectronics. 2010;**25**(5):957-966

[63] Chen Y, Nguyen A, Niu L, Corn RM. Fabrication of DNA microarrays with poly(L-glutamic acid) monolayers on gold substrates for SPR imaging measurements. Langmuir. 2009;**25**(9):5054-5060

[64] Fuchs J, Dell'Atti D, Buhot A, Calemczuk R, Mascini M, Livache T. Effects of formamide on the thermal stability of DNA duplexes on biochips. Analytical Biochemistry. 2010;**397**(1):132-134

[65] Lee HJ, Wark AW, Li Y, Corn RM. Fabricating RNA microarrays with RNA-DNA surface ligation chemistry. Analytical Chemistry. 2005;**77**(23):7832-7837

[66] Villiers MB, Cortes S, Brakha C, Marche P, Roget A, Livache T. Polypyrrole-peptide microarray for biomolecular interaction analysis by SPR imaging. Methods in Molecular Biology. 2009;**570**:317-328

[67] Bellon S, Buchmann W, Gonnet F, Jarroux N, Anger-Leroy M, Guillonneau F, et al. Hyphenation of surface plasmon resonance imaging to matrix-assisted laser desorption ionization mass spectrometry by on-chip mass spectrometry and tandem mass spectrometry analysis. Analytical Chemistry. 2009;**81**(18):7695-7702

[68] Lee HJ, Wark AW, Corn RM. Microarray methods for protein

biomarker detection. The Analyst. 2008;**133**(8):975-983

[69] Grant CF, Kanda V, Yu H, Bundle DR, McDermott MT. Optimization of immobilized bacterial disaccharides for surface plasmon resonance imaging measurements of antibody binding. Langmuir. 2008;**24**(24):14125-14132

[70] Zeidan E, Li S, Zhou Z, Miller J, Sandros MG. Single-multiplex detection of organ injury biomarkers using SPRi based nano-immunosensor. Scientific Reports. 2016;**6**:36348

[71] Hoffman IEA, Peene I, Veys EM, De Keyser F. Detection of specific antinuclear reactivities in patients with negative anti-nuclear antibody immunofluorescence screening tests. Clinical Chemistry. 2002;**48**(12):2171-2176

[72] Meroni L, Schur PH. ANA screening: An old test with new recommendations. Annals of the Rheumatic Diseases. 2010;**69**(8):1420-1422

[73] Jain A, Sharma MC, Sarkar C, Bhatia R, Singh S, Handa R. Major histocompatibility complex class I and II detection as a diagnostic tool in idiopathic inflammatory myopathies. Archives of Pathology and Laboratory Medicine. 2007;**131**(7):1070-1076

[74] Sundaram C, Uppin MS, Meena AK. Major histocompatibility complex class I expression can be used as a diagnostic tool to differentiate idiopathic inflammatory myopathies from dystrophies. Neurology India. 2008;**56**(3):363-367

[75] Van der Pas J, Hengstman GJ, ter Laak HJ, Borm GF, van Engelen BG. Diagnostic value of MHC class I staining in idiopathic inflammatory myopathies. Journal of Neurology, Neurosurgery, and Psychiatry. 2004;**75**(1):136-139

[76] Das L, Blumbergs PC, Manavis J, Limaye VS. Major histocompatibility complex class I and II expression in idiopathic inflammatory myopathy. Applied Immunohistochemistry and Molecular Morphology. 2013;**21**(6):539-542

[77] Hohlfeld R, Engel AG. The immunobiology of muscle. Immunology Today. 1994;**15**(6):269-274

[78] Nagaraju K, Casciola-Rosen L, Lundberg I, Rawat R, Cutting S, Thapliyal R, et al. Activation of the endoplasmic reticulum stress response in autoimmune myositis: Potential role in muscle fibre damage and dysfunction. Arthritis & Rheumatism. 2005;**52**(6):1824-1835

[79] Dalakas MC. Inflammatory muscle diseases: A critical review on pathogenesis and therapies. Current Opinion in Pharmacology. 2010;**10**(3):1-7

[80] Dalakas MC, Hohlfeld R. Polymyositis and dermatomyositis. Lancet. 2003;**362**(9388):971-982

[81] Civatte M, Schleinitz N, Krammer P, Fernandez C, Guis S, Veit V, et al. Class I MHC detection as a diagnostic tool in non informative muscle biopsies of patients suffering from dermatomyositis. Neuropathology and Applied Neurobiology. 2003;**29**(6):546-552

[82] Daar AS, Fuggle SV, Fabre JW, Ting A, Morris PJ. The detailed distribution of MHC class II in normal human organs. Transplantation. 1984;**38**(3):293-298

[83] Picard C, Vincent T, Lega JC, Hue S, Fortenfant F, Lakomy D, et al. Heterogeneous clinical spectrum of anti-SRP myositis and importance of the methods of detection of anti-SRP autoantibodies: A multicentric

study. Immunologic Research. 2016;**64**(3):677-686

[84] Orton SM, Peace-Brewer A, Schmitz JL, Freeman K, Miller WC, Folds JD. Practical evaluation of methods for detection and specificity of autoantibodies to extractable nuclear antigens. Clinical and Diagnostic Laboratory Immunology. 2004;**11**(2):297-301

[85] González C, Guevara P, Alarcón I, Hernando M, Navajo JA, González-Buitrago JM. Antinuclear antibodies (ANA) screening by enzyme immunoassay with nuclear HEp-2 cell extract and recombinant antigens: Analytical and clinical evaluation. Clinical Biochemistry. 2002;**35**(6):463-469

[86] Haass M, Lehmann HP. New aspects of autoantibody detection with a new combination of autoantigenic targets. Clinical and Applied Immunology Reviews. 2001;**1**(3-4):193-200

[87] Jaskowski TD, Schroder C, Martins TB, Mouritsen CL, Litwin CM, Hill HR. Screening for antinuclear antibodies by enzyme immunoassay. American Journal of Clinical Pathology. 1996;**105**(4):468-473

[88] Stinton LM, Fritzler MJ. A clinical approach to autoantibody testing in systemic autoimmune rheumatic disorders. Autoimmunity Reviews. 2007;7(1):77-84

[89] Illa I, Cortes-Vicente E, Martinez MA, Gallardo E. Diagnostic utility of cortactin antibodies in myastenia gravis. Annals of the New York Academy of Sciences. 2018;**1412**(1):90-94

[90] Shi J, Knevel R, Suwannalai P, van der Linden MP, Janssen GM, van Veelen PA, et al. Autoantibodies recognising carbamylated proteins are present in sera of patients with rheumatoid

arthritis and predict joint damage. PNAS. 2011;**108**(42):17372-17377

[91] Eissfeller P, Sticherling M, Scholz D, Hennig K, Lüttich T, Motz M, et al. Comparison of different test systems for simultaneous autoantibody detection in connective tissue diseases. Annals of the New York Academy of Sciences. 2005;**1050**:1-13

[92] Gordon P, Khamashta MA, Rosenthal E, Simpson JM, Sharland G, Brucato A, et al. Anti-52 kDa Ro, anti-60 kDa Ro, and anti-La antibody profiles in neonathal lupus. The Journal of Rheumatology. 2004;**31**(12):2480-2487

[93] Haroon N, Tsui FW, Uchanska-Ziegler B, Ziegler A, Inman RD. Endoplasmic reticulum aminopeptidase 1 (ERAP1) exhibits functionally signifi cant interaction with HLA-B27 and relates to subtype specifi city in ankylosing spondylitis. Annals of the Rheumatic Diseases. 2012;**71**(4):589-595

[94] Stagakis I, Bertsias G, Karvounaris S, Kavousanaki M, Virla D, Raptopoulou A, et al. Anti-tumor necrosis factor therapy improves insulin resistance, beta cell function and insulin signaling in active rheumatoid arthritis patients with high insulin resistance. Arthritis Research and Therapy. 2012;**14**(3):R141

[95] Tsui FWL, Tsui HW, Las Heras F, Pritzker KPH, Inman RD. Serum levels of novel noggin and sclerostin-immune complexes are elevated in ankylosing spondylitis. Annals of the Rheumatic Diseases. 2014;**73**(10):1873-1879

[96] Rizzo R, Farina I, Bortolotti D, Galuppi E, Padovan M, Di Luca D, et al. The dimeric form of HLA-G molecule is associated with the response of early rheumatoid arthritis (ERA) patients to methotrexate. Clinical Rheumatology. 2017;**36**(3):701-705

[97] Chen Z, Dodig-Crnković T, Schwenk JM, Tao S-c. Current applications of antibody microarrays. Clinical Proteomics. 2018;**15**:7

[98] Lin MW, Ho JW, Harrison LC, dos Remedios CG, Adelstein S. An antibody-based leukocyte-capture microarray for the diagnosis of systemic lupus erythematosus. PLoS One. 2013;**8**(3):e58199

[99] Carlsson A, Wuttge DM, Ingvarsson J, Bengtsson AA, Sturfelt G, Borrebaeck CA, et al. Serum protein profiling of systemic lupus erythematosus and systemic sclerosis using recombinant antibody microarrays. Molecular and Cellular Proteomics. 2011;**10**(5):M110.005033

[100] Schumacher S, Muekusch S, Seitz H. Up-to-date applications of microarrays and their way to commercialization. Microarrays (Basel). 2015;**4**(2):196-213

[101] Charpin C, Arnoux F, Martin M, Toussirot E, Lambert N, Balandraud N, et al. New autoantibodies in early rheumatoid arthritis. Arthritis Research and Therapy. 2013;**15**(4):R78

[102] Abel L, Kutschki S, Turewicz M, Eisenacher M, Stoutjesdijk J, Meyer HE, et al. Autoimmune profiling with protein microarrays in clinical applications. Biochimica et Biophysica Acta. 2014;**1844**(5):9779-9787

[103] Sajda T, Hazelton J, Patel M, Seiffert-Sinha K, Steinman L, Robinson W, et al. Multiplexed autoantigen microarrays identify HLA as a key driver of anti-desmoglein and -non-desmoglein reactivities in pemphigus. PNAS. 2016;**113**(7):1859-1864

[104] Kim YG, Sohn DH, Zhao X, Sokolove J, Lindstrom TM, Yoo B, et al. Role of protein phosphatase magnesium-dependent 1A and

anti-protein phosphatase magnesium-dependent 1A autoantibodiesin ankylosing spondylitis. Arthritis & Rheumatism. 2014;**66**(10):2793-2803

[105] Gonzalez C, Garcia-Berrocal B, Talavan T, Cassas ML, Navajo JA, Gonzalez-Buitargo JM. Clinical evaluation of a microsphere bead-based flow cytometry assay for the simultaneous determination of anti thyroid peroxidase and anti thyroglobulin antibodies. Clinical Biochemistry. 2005;**38**(11):966-972

[106] Gonzales-Buitrago JM. Multiplexed testing in the autoimmunity laboratory. Clinical Chemistry and Laboratory Medicine. 2006;**44**(10):1169-1174

[107] Rouquete AM, Desgruelles C, Laroche P. Evaluation of the new multiplexed immunoassay, FIDIS, for simultaneous quantitative determination of antinuclear antibodies and comparison with conventional methods. American Journal of Clinical Pathology. 2003;**120**(5):676-681

[108] Feng Y, Ke X, Ma R, Chen Y, Hu G, Liu F. Parallel detection of autoantibodies with microarray in rheumatoid diseases. Clinical Chemistry. 2004;**50**(2):416-422

[109] Fritzler MJ. Advances and applications of multiplexed diagnostic technologies in autoimmune diseases. Lupus. 2006;**15**(7):422-427

[110] Seideman J, Peritt D. A novel monoclonal antibody screening method using the Luminex-100 microsphere system. Journal of Immunological Methods. 2002;**267**(2):165-171

[111] Mattey DL, Packham JC, Nixon NB, Coates L, Creamer P, Hailwood S, et al. Association of cytokine and matrix metalloproteinase profiles with disease activity and function in ankylosing spondylitis. Arthritis Research and Therapy. 2012;**14**(3):R127

[112] Limon-Camacho L, Vargas-Rojas MI, Velasquez-Mellardo J, Casasola-Vargas J, Moctezuma JF, Burgos-Vargas R, et al. *In vivo* peripheral blood proinflammatory T cells in patients with ankylosing spondylitis. Journal of Rheumatology. 2012;**39**(4):830-835

[113] Mou Y, Wu Z, Gu J, Liao Z, Lin Z, Wei Q, et al. HLA-B27 polymorphism in patients with juvenile and adult-onset ankylosing spondylitis in Southern China. Tissue Antigens. 2010;**75**(1):56-60

[114] Lokate AMC, Beusink JB, Besselink GAJ, Pruijn GJM, Schasfoort RBM. Biomolecular interaction monitoring of autoantibodies by scanning surface plasmon resonance microarray imaging. Journal of the American Chemical Society. 2007;**129**(45):14013-14018

[115] van Beers JBC, Willemze A, Jansen JJ, Engbers GHM, Salden M, Raats J, et al. ACPA fine-specificity profiles in early rheumatoid arthritis patients do not correlate with clinical features at baseline or with disease progression. Arthritis Research and Therapy. 2013;**15**(5):R140

[116] van Beers JJ, Raijmakers R, Alexander LE, Stammen-Vogelzangs J, Lokate AM, Heck AJ, et al. Mapping of citrullinated fibrinogen B-cell epitopes in rheumatoid arthritis by imaging surface plasmon resonance. Arthritis Research and Therapy. 2010;**12**(6):R219

[117] Martinez-Perdiguero J, Retolaza A, Bujanda L, Merino S. Surface plasmon resonance immunoassay for the detection of theTNFα biomarker in human serum. Talanta. 2014;**119**:492-497

[118] Buhl A, Metzger JH, Heegaard NH, von Landenberg P, Flek M, Luppa PB. Novel biosensorbased analytic device for the detection of

anti-double-stranded DNA antibodies. Clinical Chemistry. 2007;**53**(2):334-341

[119] Vergani D, Alvarez F, Bianchi FB, Cancado ELR, Mackay IR, Manns MP, et al. Liver autoimmune serology: A consesus statement from the committee for autoimmune serology of the International Autoimmune Hepatitis Group. Journal of Hepatology. 2004;**41**(4):677-683

[120] Törn C, Mueller P, Schlosser M, Bonifacio E, Bingley P. Diabetes Antibody Standardization Program: Evaluation of assays for autoantibodies to glutamic acid decarboxylase and islet antigen-2. Diabetologia. 2008;**51**(5):846-852

[121] Hayashi N, Kawamoto T, Mukai M, Morinobu A, Koshiba M, Kondo S, et al. Detection of antinuclear antibodies by use of an enzyme immunoassay with nuclear HEp-2 cell extract and recombinant antigens: Comparison with immunofluorescence assay in 307 patients. Clinical Chemistry. 2001;**47**(9):1649-1659

[122] Fenger M, Wiik A, Høter-Madsen M, Lykkegaard JJ, Rozenfeld T, Hansen MS, et al. Detection of antinuclear antibodies by solid-phase immunoassays and immunofluorescence analysis. Clinical Chemistry. 2004;**50**(11):2141-2147

[123] Tozzoli R, Bizzaro N, Tonutti E, Pradella M, Manoni F, Vilalta D, et al. Immunoassay of anti-thyroid autoantibodies: High analytical variability in second generation methods. Clinical Chemistry and Laboratory Medicine. 2002;**40**(6):568-573

[124] Fritzler MJ, Behmanesh F, Fritzler ML. Analysis of human sera that are polyreactive in an addressable laser bead immunoassay. Clinical Immunology. 2006;**120**(3):349-356

[125] Nifli AP, Notas G, Mamoulaki M, Niniraki M, Ampartzaki V, Theodoropoulos PA, et al. Comparison of a multiplex, bead-based fluorescent assay and immunofluorescence methods for the detection of ANA and ANCA autoantibodies in human serum. Journal of Immunological Methods. 2006;**311**(1-2):189-197

[126] Biagini RE, Parks CG, Smith JP, Sammons DL, Robertson SA. Analytical performance of the AtheNA MultiLyte ANAII assay in sera from lupus patients with multiple positive ANAs. Analytical and Bioanalytical Chemistry. 2007;**388**(3):613-618

[127] Avaniss-Aghajani E, Berzon S, Sarkissian A. Clinical value of multiplex bead based immunoassay for detection of autoantibodies to nuclear antigens. Clinical and Vaccine Immunology. 2007;**14**(5):505-509

[128] Salamunić I, Pauković-Sekulić B, Galetović A, Tandara L, Martinović-Kaliterna D. Comparative analysis of multiplex AtheNA Multi-Lyte ANA test system and conventional laboratory methods to detect autoantibodies. Biochemia Medica. 2008;**18**(1):88-98

[129] Elshal MF, McCoy JP. Multiplex bead array assays: Performance evaluation and comparison of sensitivity to ELISA. Methods. 2006;**38**(4):317-323

Chapter 5

Immunogenetic and Immunotherapy in Tuberculosis

Gloria Guillermina Guerrero Manriquez

Abstract

Tuberculosis (TB) is an infectious disease caused by *Mycobacterium tuberculosis* (MTb). TB causes mortality of millions of people every year. *Mycobacterium bovis Bacillus Calmette Güerin* (BCG) is the only officially approved vaccine that protects against miliary TB and children but fails to protect in adulthood presumably because of the lack of long lasting immunological memory. The problem is even more aggravated because of the emergence of multidrug-resistant strains. Therefore, immunogenetics and immunotherapy of antimycobacterial immunity are complex and poorly characterized. However, several studies either in the mouse model or *in vitro*, using derived dendritic or macrophages derived from PBMCs or human cell lines, have shown that Th1 type cellular immune response represented by IFN-γ, IL-12 in conjunction with IL-17, and IL-23 are key players of the immune protection to M. *tuberculosis*. It is known that under different settings type I IFNs promote bacterial virulence and disease exacerbation, since a study with active TB patients was concomitant with a dominant neutrophil-driven interferon inducible gene pattern. Furthermore, in an independent cohort of TB patients, ex vivo experiments with BMDCs (bone marrow–derived dendritic cells) and myeloid from lung showed that there is a cross action between the components of IL-1β, eicosanoid pathways (prostaglandin, lipoxins, and leukotrienes) in active TB, while excessive type I IFNs and IL10 induction, concomitant with an inhibition of iNO3 and prostaglandin, could be found. These responses could be used as a therapeutic target instead of any other treatment based on antibiotics. Furthermore, the work from us has demonstrated that interferon alpha plus BCG vaccine protects against mycobacterial infections through modulating the Th1-type cellular immune response, iNOs, and IL-1β production. These immunomodulatory properties of interferon alpha could influence the outcome of the innate and acquired host immune responses in tuberculosis.

Keywords: type I IFNs, adjuvants, *mycobacterial* infections, BCG vaccine, Th1-type cytokines, IL17, iNOS3

1. Introduction

Tuberculosis is the most serious cause of mortality after HIV/AIDS [1, 2]. Until now, BCG is the only officially approved vaccine that protects against miliary TB in children but it fails to protect in adulthood [1–3]. Therefore, the search for subunits agents that can boost primarily the central memory is still an issue of intense research worldwide [1, 2]. Several candidates have been developed and are under clinical studies [4–8]. Type I IFNs emerge, thus, as a

IntechOpen

potential candidate adjuvant in bacterial infections. More than half century ago, interferons were first described like an antiviral "activity" [9–12]. Later on, they were recognized as innate inflammatory cytokines, and considered to be major connector of the innate and adaptive immunity. In general, type I IFNs could be considered like pleiotropic cytokines that belong to a multigenic family as outlined in **Table 1** [11, 12].

Plasmacytoid dendritic cells (pDCs) are known to be major producers of type I IFNs producing up to hundred to a thousand times more IFNs-α than other cell types [13, 14]. To be produced, a recognition between pathogen-associated molecular patterns (PAMPs) on the pathogen surface (viral and bacterial), Toll-like receptors (TLRs) (bacterial), with the pattern recognition receptor (PRRs), antigen-presenting cells (dendritic cells and macrophages) is necessary; followed by the activation of Myd88, interferon regulatory factor 3 (IRF3), IRF5 and IRF7 (IFN-α), and NFκβ [13, 15]. Except leucocytes (which produce primarily IFN sub-types), all cells are capable of detecting intracellular PAMPs and producing IFN-β following activation of IRF3 and NF-κβ [14, 16]. After viral or bacterial infections, there is an increase in the IFNs production in different types of cells. The functions *in vivo* of type I IFNs are the activation of DCs (dendritic cells), critical antigen-presenting cell for initiating immunity [13], in fact, type I IFN-treated DCs prime T cells *in vitro* promote the expression of costimulatory molecules [15], stimulate human blood monocytes differentiation into DCs [15]. Regardless of its role as an antiviral agent [11, 12], type I IFNs are also able to enhance adaptive immunity. A huge body of studies have shown type I IFNs immunomodulatory properties either to virus as well as to bacteria infections [12–15]. We think in agreement with other groups that type I IFNs have a strikingly dichotomy behavior, since their actions can be either positive or negative depending on the settings and the surrounding scenery that will strongly influence the outcome of the host immune response.

IFNs I 17 sub-types	IFNs II	IFNs III 4 sub-types
All nucleated cells	Immune cells	Epithelial cells
α /β		
α: 12 genes Ifn-β (PBMCs) Ifn-ε (genital tract) Ifn-κ(keratinocytes	IFN-Y	(IFN-λs) IFN-λsI IFN-λsII
Ifn-ω Ifn-ζ (mice and rrophoblastic) Ifn-τ (ungulates) Ifn-δ (pigs)		IFN-λsIII IFN-λsIV

Table 1.
The multigenic family of type I IFNs in nature.

2. The type I IFNs in nature

As outlined in **Table 1**, several human type I IFNs are already known to be selectively produced in a tissue-specific. As a multigenic family, type I IFNs, in particular, IFN-alpha, are comprised of 13, while IFN-β, IFN-ε (genital tract), IFN-κ (keratinocytes), and IFN-ω are only coded for a single gene. For the signalization to be carried out, there are basically two main steps that are common to the 17 IFNs. First is the binding to and signal through a shared heterodimeric receptor complex composed of a single chain of IFNAR1 and IFNAR2, which is present in almost on all nucleated cells [13–15]. Second, a signal is propagated within the cell via the JAK-STAT signaling pathway [13–15]. This is also common to type III IFNs. As occurred in other interaction receptor-ligand, there are low or high affinity binding, and this could impact in the stability and the variety of the complex formed and therefore in the outcome of the host response [13–15]. This point has been the focus of intense research, because many questions arise for this interaction. Thus, for example, it is intriguing: why some interferons signal through the same receptor? Is there a redundancy of the immune system or is tailoring for each type of pathogen? Is the molecular evolution that has an impact also in the transcriptional gene printing, or in the adjuvant activities?

One of the hallmarks of the IFN action in nature is its immunomodulatory behavior [7, 10, 17]. These include among others the role of type I IFNs in the connection of innate and adaptive immune responses, such as B activation for enhancement of Ab responses [7, 10, 18], promotion of Th1 responses in terms of IgG2a Ab production, and CD4 + T cells activation and induction of an *in vitro* and *in vivo* differentiation of monocytes into functionally active DC [8, 19, 20], NK and T cytolytic activity, upregulation of histocompatibility antigen class I expression, induction of proliferation, and long-term survival of memory CD8 + T cells [7, 19, 20].

3. Is there any specificity in the type I IFN induction?

At glance yes, it would seem that there is specificity in the type I IFNs induction. As highlighted above, type I IFNs induction is a consequence of the host-pathogen interaction [10, 16]. Thus, while membrane-bound PRRs are endowed with the ability to recognize viral or bacterial PAMPS (located in the cell surface, and within endosomal compartments [20]), it could be possible that the expression profile of each cell type in particular of these PRRS on the innate immune cells that could potentially give rise to specificity in IFN subtype production—an early step during infection inward ultimately fine-tuning the immune response—an issue that is challenging because to measure the different profiles of IFN-α for each cell type has enormous limitations under physiological conditions, but it is true that should be pinpointed whether the IFN responses are qualitatively different in response to distinct pathogens [9, 20]. Furthermore, IFN-β and/or the IFN-α subtypes signal through TLRs (TLRs are membrane-bound compartments) of cosmopolitan expression in different human cells, which can potentially give some specificity to the interaction. Thus, it is known from the literature that TLR3, TLR7, TLR8, and TLR9 recognize viral nucleic acids [9, 10, 16]. Another type of receptor, specialized in detecting pathogen-derived RNA in the cytoplasm, that is also involved in the production of IFN-β in nonimmune cells, is the members of the RIG-I-like receptors (RLRs), a family of cytoplasmic RNA helicases important for host viral responses and includes retinoic acid-inducible gene I (RIG-I)-melanoma differentiation-associated protein 5 (MDA5) and the laboratory of genetics and physiology-2-(LGP3). The signalization through these receptors initiates via these intracellular PRRS set in motion a series of events that has resulted in IRF3 and NF-κβ activation, both of which are required for the production of IFN-β and the release of chemokines that recruit immune cells to the site of infection [7, 9, 16].

4. How type I IFNs become central players in the connection between innate and acquired immune response

Type I IFNs are the dominant player of the connection between the innate and adaptive immune responses through the main interaction with antigen-presenting immune cells, such as dendritic cells (DCs), in particular, with plasmacytoid dendritic cells (pDCs) [6, 18, 21], which are precisely the major producers of type I IFNs producing up to a hundred to a thousand times more IFNs-α than other cell types [13, 14]. This is supported from *in vitro* experiments that have shown that type I IFN-treated DCs prime T cells *in vitro* more effectively [11, 12, 15].

5. How to calibrate host immune response to bacterial infections?

Calibrating host immune system for bacterial infections initiated as outlined above through the surface membrane conserved molecules organized in "patterns" such as peptidoglycan (PGN), lipopolysaccharide (LPS), and nucleic acid structures or pathogen-associated molecular patterns (PAMPs). Whereas, innate cells have the counterpart, "PRRS" (pattern recognition pathogen) [8, 10, 16], that automatically unlock the unspecificity of the type I IFNs production, the recognition of the "self" versus "nonself" [9], one PRRS for a particular type of PAMPs either bacterial, fungal, or virus; followed by a more general signalization route through Myd88 and IRFs (this could be also specific for each type of IFNs), and finally, NF-κβ translocation to the nucleus and thus IFNs production [8–10]. The synthesis of type I IFNs is not the job of a specialized cell type. However, an important distinction must be made between those cells that produce just enough type I IFNs to affect the local environment, and those produced by IFN-producing cells (IPCs) which could contribute to connect innate and adaptive immune responses more effectively. How much is produced or how much should be produced depends mostly on the tissue involved and the signal received, in particular, viral, bacterial [6, 18, 21]. Therefore, it is intriguing that all IFN-α proteins interact with the same receptor complex and have a spectrum of distinct effects, that goes from the specific antiviral capacity of individual IFN-α to differences in the activation of natural killer (NK) cells [16, 17]. Trying to understand why some types of IFNs, one temptative explanation could be, different temporal or spatial regulation of their expression, which might impact in the molecular calibration of the host immune response to viral or bacterial infections since TLR signaling targets (such as NF-κβ) and IFNAR signaling targets (such as STAT) converge at their promoters [10, 16]. Thus, it seems possible to think that it is the TLR4 signaling that arises as a key player for type I IFNs production by different cell types in response to Gram-negative pathogens. Several studies have in addition highlighted this point, some has been concentrated in the LPS effect [8, 16] on the type I IFNS induction, while others have focused in the gene that encode inducible oxide nitric synthase (iNOS), which is more evident once a bacterial signal through TLR, as demonstrated with Chlamydia spp. [8, 16]. Despite this gap in our knowledge, the gene encoding iNOs is a paradigm for antimicrobial genes requiring type I IFN synthesis and expression downstream of TLR, implying a potential important role of type I IFN synthesis during nonviral infection. More recent infection studies that have investigated the mechanism behind this type I IFN effect demonstrated its importance in generating TNF-α, Il-1β, or bacterial signals (Chlamydia spp). IL-12-independent cellular immunity to *S. typhimurium*. This was attributed to the ability of type I IFNs to stimulate STAT-4 tyrosine phosphorylation in NK cells and Th1 cells. Together with IL-18 signals, this triggers expression of the IFN-alpha gene [8, 16]. In addition, it has been described that the induction of intrinsic immunity to kill bacteria or prevent their invasion and the regulation of chemokines, proinflammatory cytokines, and phagocytic cells. The mechanism by which IFN-α/β promotes host protective responses or susceptibility in bacterial pathogens is poorly defined and the factors that determine whether a response will be protective or pathogenic are not yet fully understood. However, it is well known that type I IFNs that are released during bacterial infection by IFN-producing cells (IPDCs) can cause the activation of signal transducer and activator of transcription 4 (STAT 4) in natural killer (NK) and T helper (TH1 cells) [5, 8, 10, 16]. In conjunction with interleukin 18 (IL-18)-derived signals, STAT-4 stimulates the expression of the IFN-alpha genes, which provide antibacterial immunity, such as macrophage activation [22, 23]. In addition, type I IFNs make important contributions to the maturation and activation of dendritic ells (DCs) [24], and in this way, influence antigen presentation, T cell activation, and the development of adaptive immune responses.

6. Dichotomy in the type I IFNs' action in bacterial infections

In contrast to viral infections, IFN-α/β can be protective or can have detrimental effects for the host during bacterial infections in a bacterium-specific manner, although less is known about the role of these. By one side, IFN-α/β-mediated signaling primes the production of interleukin-10 (IL-10), proinflammatory cytokines, and antimicrobial effector mechanism. But, IL-10 mediates a negative feedback loop, suppressing the production of proinflammatory cytokine, including IL-12, tumor necrosis factor (TNF), and IL-1 α/β cytokines that are key in the host resistance to bacterial infections. Moreover, some studies have addressed to decreased bacterial load and/or improved host survival in the absence of IFN-α/β-mediated signaling. Thus, for example, IFN-α/β contributes to priming the host to clear the virus, while increasing host susceptibility to bacterial assault. Interestingly, under this scenario, IFN-α/β produced in response to infections is damaging to the host but would normally be protecting during a primary infection, i.e., *S. pneumoniae* or *E. coli* [8, 10, 16]. This would imply that the circumstances of IFN-α/β production and action are crucial to determine host protection versus pathogenesis and highlight also the dichotomy role of IFN-α/β depending on the pathogen. These different issues have been pinpointed and clearly showed that, for example, on mycobacterial infections, there is a detrimental effect of type I IFNs in active TB patient, which showed in blood a remarkable transcriptional gene expression profile in neutrophils that correlated with extensive lesion in lung [25]. In a different cohort of patients from Africa, it was also found that this same result, the broad signature of IFN-α/β, could be found anywhere [25]. These findings have revealed the dark side of these cytokines that is—the ability to suppress host immune protective response by downregulating the Th1-type cellular immune responses (IFN-gamma IL12 production), iNOS3 synthesis while inducing IL-10. In summary, favorable or unfavorable effect can be determined by the infecting strain, the severity of infection, the stage of infection, and the interplay among the different immune effector mechanisms.

7. Signalization pathways of type I IFNs as an adjuvant

Adjuvants can stimulate innate immunity by interacting with specialized pattern recognition receptors (PRRs) including Toll-like receptors (TLRs) [26, 27] and nucleotide-binding oligomerization domain receptors [28]. These PRRs are immersed in the membrane surface of the antigen presenting such as DCs or macrophages, even in epithelial and B cells. Once this interaction is initiated, it is followed by serial reactions that lead to the production of proinflammatory cytokines and chemokines that will influence drastically the outcome of the host immune response. The shape of this response will be affected by initial stimulus, and therefore, the antigen-presenting cells (M1, M2) as well as the T cell population will adopt a state of differentiation (Th1/Th2/Th3) [29]. However, many cell types, including nonhematopoietic cells, express PRR and produce cytokines during innate immunity [30]. In conjunction, adjuvant action could be viewed as the contribution of cytokines milieu and the different cellular sources of them in order to initiate and potentiate immunity from the native polyclonal repertoire cells and molecules.

The role of IFN-I as natural immune adjuvants for commercial vaccines [18, 21, 31] was established by showing that either mucosal or intramuscular administration of influenza virus antigen-admixed IFN-I to mice enhances viral resistance and increased production of antiviral Ab [18, 21]. The adjuvant activity of IFN-I leads to potentiate the adaptive immune response by directly stimulating lymphocytes or activating DC that represents the critical antigen-presenting cells governing the fate of helper T cell responses [18, 21, 24, 25]. The immunity-promoting activity of IFN-I can result from a direct effect on T cells. In this situation, IFN-I acts as "third signal" of activation, helping to sustain survival of proliferating cells. IFN-I also supports Th1 differentiation, activation of STAT-4 signaling, and IFN-γ production [24, 25]. These activities are reminiscent of the biological effects of IL-12 and could have a role in the observed adjuvant type I IFN activities. Indeed, the variable need for IFN-I to act directly on T cells during activation and differentiation may thus arise from a similarly variable production of IL-12.

8. How type I IFNs shape the host immune system to antimycobacterial infection?

Despite the wealth of studies, shaping the host immune response to bacterial infection is complex and still remains to be characterized. Type I IFNs can shape the antimycobacterial immunity by enhancing action of dendritic cells and monocytes, by promoting CD4+ and Cd8 T cell responses, by enhancing NK cell responses and B cell responses [8, 10, 16, 18, 21]. Type I IFNs (IFN-α/β) have a direct effect on the maturation of DCs, through increasing cell surface expression of MHC molecules as well as costimulatory molecules such as CD80 and CD86, leading to an augmented activation of T cells. Another effect of type I IFNs (IFN-α/β) is to promote the migration of DCs to lymph nodes through upregulating chemokine receptor expression thus promoting T cell activation. Moreover, direct downregulation of IFN-γR expression may not be the central mechanism by which IFN-αβ exerts their effects on IFN-γ activity [7–10, 18, 21–23], instead, in both mouse and human cells, it has been shown that IFN-αβ potently suppresses the ability of macrophages to upregulate antimycobacterial effector molecules and to restrict bacterial growth, in response to both *M. leprae* and *M tuberculosis*. The importance of this mechanism of action of IFN-αβ is further suggested by experiment using Ifngr 1-/- or Ifnar1-/- mice, which suggests that IFN-αβ contributes to host protection in the absence of the IFN-γ pathway [16, 17, 22, 23]. In another study, it was observed a natural mutation in the gene ISG15 in humans that conferred host-protective response mediated by type I IFNs (IFN-αβ) *to M. tuberculosis* infection [23]. No further studies were made. Similarly, it has been reported that IL-12p70 suppressed type I IFNs (IFN-αβ) during *M. tuberculosis* infection [27, 28, 32]. This suppression could result from the presence of IL-10, the downregulation of IFN-γR, and/or the induction of negative regulators of IFN-mediated signaling such as protein arginine methyltransferase-1(PRMT1) [9, 10, 21, 22]. Finally, IFN-αβ, possibly by influencing chemokine expression, has been shown to be involved in the generation and trafficking of *M. tuberculosis* permissive innate cells to the lungs in a mouse model thus contributing to the exacerbation of infection [8, 9, 26, 31, 32].

Several human clinical studies have obtained favorable assessment of using aerosolized IFN-α as adjuvant therapy for patients with tuberculosis [33]. However, it has been shown that there is a TB reactivation during IFN-alpha treatment for hepatitis D infection [33]. In a different study, it has been also demonstrated that in active TB patients, there is a correlation between the extent of lung lesion with the transcriptional signature of type I IFNs in blood, in particular, in neutrophils [25]. This was also found in a cohort of Africa and Indonesia. These findings implied that the type I IFNs are common broad signature and strengthened the role of these cytokines in the pathogenesis of TB [8, 9, 25, 26, 34]. Indeed, seminal work by Giacomini et al., [24] have demonstrated that IFN-β improves *M. bovis* BCG vaccine immunogenic capacity by exerting a strong influence of DCs maturation, throughout enhancing costimulatory molecules such as CD86, CD83, and therefore, increased IL-12 which will act on macrophage killing activities [18, 20, 29, 30]. Later on, further studies by Mayer-Babier et al. [34] have demonstrated that the action of type I IFNs in tuberculosis could reside in the pathways of IL-1β, arachidonic acids, prostaglandins, and iNOs. Active TB patients showed an increased production of these molecules. This constitutes the first cue for a clinical therapeutic target of TB [34]. In more recent work by us, we found that type I IFNs action, in particular, interferon alpha, could exert its action in conjunction with *M. bovis* BCG vaccine that potentially could be signaling through Toll-like receptor and/or tentative through IFN-R1, leading to a protective antimycobacterial immune response, i.e., Th1-type cytokines and so far to IL-17 and IL23 production [35–37].

Author details

Gloria Guillermina Guerrero Manriquez
Immunobiology Laboratory, Science Biological Unit, Autonome University of
Zacatecas, Zacatecas, Mexico

*Address all correspondence to: gloguerrero9@gmail.com

IntechOpen

© 2019 The Author(s). Licensee IntechOpen. This chapter is distributed under the terms
of the Creative Commons Attribution License (http://creativecommons.org/licenses/
by/3.0), which permits unrestricted use, distribution, and reproduction in any medium,
provided the original work is properly cited. (cc) BY

References

[1] WHO. *World Health Organization: Tuberculosis—Global Facts 2011/2102.* Geneva: WHO Stop TB Department; 2012. http://www.who.int/tb/publications/2011/factsheet_tb_2011.pdf

[2] Maher D, Raviglione M. Global epidemiology of tuberculosis. Clinics in Chest Medicine. 2005;**26**:167-182

[3] Rodriguez LC, Diwan VK, Wheeler JG. Protective effect of BCG against tuberculosis meningitis and military tuberculosis: A metaanalysis. International Journal of Epidemiology. 1993;**22**:1154-1158

[4] Young DB, Perkins MD, Duncan K, Barry CE III. Confornting the scientific obstacle to global control of tuberculosis. The Journal of clinical investigation. 2008;**118**:1255-1265

[5] Andersen P, Doherty TM. The success and failure of BCG-implications for a novel tuberculosis vaccine. Nature Reviews Microbiology. 2005;**3**:656-662

[6] Nolz JC, Harty JT. Strategies and implications for prime-boost vaccination to generate memory CD8+ T cells. Adv. Exp. Med. Biol. 2011;**780**:69-83

[7] Skeiky YAW, JC Sadoff. Advances in tuberculosis vaccine strategies. Nature Reviews Microbiology. 2006;**4**:469-476

[8] Roediger EK, Kugathasan K, Zhang X, Lichty BD, Xing Z. Heterologous boosting of recombinant adenoviral prime immunization with a novel vesicular stomatitis virus-vectored tuberculosis vaccine. Molecular Therapy. 2008;**16**:1161-1169

[9] O'Garra A, Redford SP, McNab WF, Bloom ICH, Wilkinson JR, Perry MPR. The immune response in tuberculosis. Annual Review of Immunology. 2013;**31**:475-527

[10] Cooper AM. Cell-mediated immune responses in tuberculosis. Annual Review of Immunology. 2009;**27**:393-422

[11] Ferrantini M, Capone I, Belardelli F. Interferon-alpha/beta and cancer: Mechanisms of actions and new perspectives of clinical use. Biochimie. 2007;**89**:884-893

[12] González-Navajas JM, Lee J, David M, Raz E. Immunomodulatory functions of type I interferons. Nature Reviews. Immunology. 2012;**12**:125-135

[13] Decker T, Müller M, Stockinger S. The Yin and Yang of type I interfron activity in bacterial infection. Nature Reviews Immunology. 2005;**5**:675-687. DOI: 101038/nri1684

[14] Hoffmann HH, Schneider MW, MCh R. Interferons and viruses: An evolutionary arms race of molecular interactions. Cell. Trends in Immunology. 2015;**36**:124-138

[15] McNab F, Mayer-Barber K, Sher A, Wack A, O'Garra A. Type I interferon in infectious disease. Nature Reviews Immunology. 2015;**15**:67-103

[16] Decker T, Stockinger S, Karagbiosoff M, Müller M, Kovanik P. IFNs and STATs in innate immunity to microorganism. The Journal of Clinical Investigation. 2002;**109**:1271-1277

[17] Travar M, Petkovic M, Verhza A. Type I, II and III interferons: Regulating immunity to M. tuberculosis infection. Archivum Immunologiae et Therapiae Experimentalis. 2015;**64**:19-31. DOI: 10.1007. 00005-015-0365

[18] Couch RB, Atmar RL, Cate TR, Quarles JM, Keitel WA, Arden NH, et al. Contrasting effects of type I interferon as a mucosal adjuvant for influenza

vaccine in mice and humans. Vaccine. 2009;**27**:5344-5348

[19] Prchal M, Pilz A, Simma O, Lingnau K, von Gabain A, Strobl B, et al. Type I interferon as mediators of immune adjuvants for T and B cell dependent acquired immunity. Vaccine. 2009;**275**:G17-G20

[20] Cooper AM, Mayer-Barber KD, Sher A. Role of the innate-cytokine in mycobacterial infections. Mucosal Immunology. 2011;**4**:252-260

[21] Desvignes L, Wolf AJ, Ernst JD. Dynamic roles of type I and type II IFNs in early infection with *Mycobacterium tuberculosis*. Journal of Immunology. 2012;**188**:6205-6215

[22] Teles MBR, Graeber GT, Krutzik RS, Montoya D, Schenk M, Lee JD, et al. Type I interferon suppresses type II interferon-triggered human anti-mycobacterial responses. Science. 2013;**339**:1448-1453

[23] Giacomini E, Remoli ME, Gata V, Pardini M, Fattorini L, Coccia EM. IFN-β improves immunogenicity by acting on DC maturation. Journal of Leukocyte Biology. 2009;**85**:462-468

[24] Berry PRM, Graham MC, McNab WF, Xu Z, Bloch AAS, Oni T, et al. An interferon-inducible neutrophil-driven blood transcriptional signature in human tuberculosis. Nature. 2010;**466**:973-979

[25] Ho HH, Ivashkiv LB. Role of STAT-3 in type I interferon responses. Negative regulation of STAT1-dependent inflammatory gene activation. The Journal of Biological Chemistry. 2006;**281**:14111-14118

[26] Manca C, Tsenova L, Freeman S, Barczak AK, Tovey M, Murray PJ, et al. Hypervirulent *M. tuberculosis* W/ Beijing strains upregulate type I IFNs

and increase expression of negative regulators of the Jak-Stat pathway. Journal of Interferon & Cytokine Research. 2005;**25**:694-701

[27] Manca C, Tsenova L, Bergtold A, Freeman SH, Tovey M, Musser MJ, et al. Virulence of a *Mycobacterium tuberculosis* clinical isolate in mice is determined by failure to induce Th1 type immunity and is associated with induction of IFN-α/β. Proceedings of the National Academy of Sciences. 2007;**98**:5752-5757

[28] O'Shea JJ, Visconti R. Type I IFNs and regulation of TH1 responses: Enigmas both resolved and emerge. Nature Immunology. 2000;**1**:17-19

[29] Bracci L, Canini I, Puzelli S, Sestili P, Venditti M, Spleda M, et al. Type I IFN is a powerful mucosal adjuvant for a selective intranasal vaccination against influenza virus in mice and affects antigen capture at mucosal level. Vaccine. 2005;**23**:2994-3004

[30] Longhi PM, Trumpfheller C, Idoyaga J, Caskey M, Matos I, Kluger C, et al. Dendritic cells require a systemic type I interferon response to mature and induce CD4+ Th1 immunity with poly IC as adjuvant. The Journal of Experimental Medicine. 2011;**208**:1589-1802

[31] Zhang D, Zhang D-E. Interferon-stimulated gene 15 and the protein ISGylation system. Journal of Interferon & Cytokine Research. 2011;**31**:119-130. DOI: 10.1089/jir. 2010.0110

[32] Feng C, Jankovic D, Kulberg M, Cheever A, Scanga C, Hieny S, et al. Maintenance of pulmonary Th1 effector function in chronic tuberculosis requires persistent IL-12 production. Journal of Immunology. 2005;**174**:4185-4192

[33] Mayer-Barber DK, Andrade BB, Oland DS, Amaral PE, Barber ID, Gonzalez J, et al. Host-directed therapy

of tuberculosis based on interleukin-1 and type I interferon crosstalk. Nature. 2014;**511**:99-115

[34] Telesca C, Angelico M, Piccolo P, Nosotti L, Morrone A, Longhi C, et al. Interferon–alpha treatment of hepatitis D induces tuberculosis exacerbation in an immigrant. The Journal of Infection. 2007;**54**:e223-e226

[35] Ottenhoff TH, Dass RH, Yang N, Zhang MM, Wong HE, Sahiratmadja E, et al. Genome-wide expression profiling identified type 1 interferon response pathways in active tuberculosis. PLoS One. 2012;7:e45839

[36] Guerrero GG, Rangel-Moreno J, Islas Trujillo I, Espinosa-Rojas O. Successive intramuscular boosting with IFN-alpha to BCG vaccinated mice protects against *M. lepraemurium*. BioMed Research International. 2015; **2015**:1-9. DOI: 10.1155/2015/414027

[37] Rivas Santiago C, Guerrero GG. IFN-α boosting of *Mycobacterium bovis Bacillus Calmette Güerin* (BCG)-vaccine promoted Th1 type cellular response and protect *against M. tuberculosis infection*. BioMed Research International. 2017;**2017**:1-8

www.ingramcontent.com/pod-product-compliance
Lightning Source LLC
Chambersburg PA
CBHW081236190326
41458CB00016B/5805